simple
massage

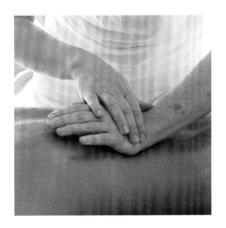

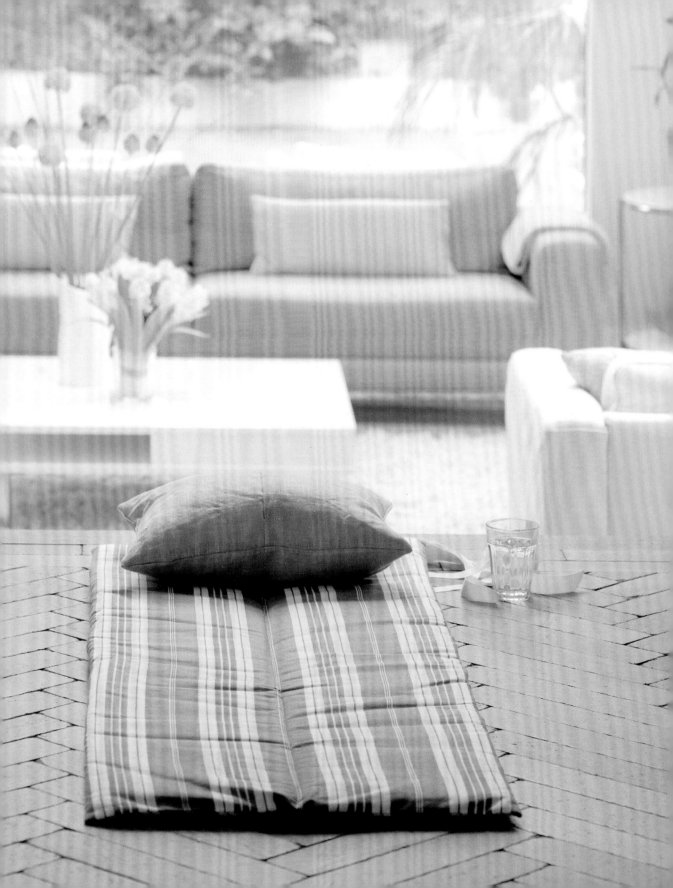

simple massage

TECHNIQUES FOR RELAXATION, HEALING, AND EMPOWERMENT

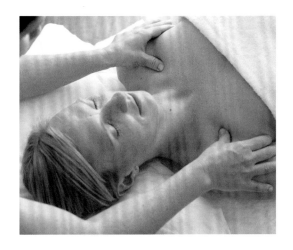

DAPHNE ROUBINI

CICO BOOKS

LONDON NEW YORK

To my late dad, Samuel Roubini

This edition published in 2024 by CICO Books,
an imprint of Ryland Peters & Small Ltd

20–21 Jockey's Fields
London WC1R 4BW

341 E 116th St
New York, NY 10029

www.rylandpeters.com

First published in 2007 as *Healing Massage*.

A CIP catalogue record for this book is available from
the Library of Congress and the British Library.

ISBN: 978-1-80065-338-2

Printed in China

Step-by-step photography by Tino Tedaldi.
For other picture credits, see page 144

Editor: Richard Emerson
Designer: Geoff Borin
Art director: Sally Powell
Creative director: Leslie Harrington
Head of production: Patricia Harrington
Publishing manager: Carmel Edmonds

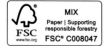

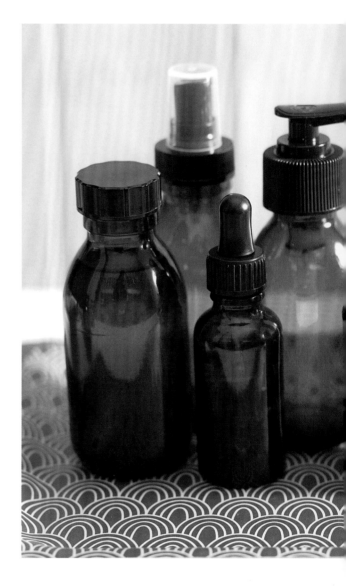

Publisher's note:
Always consult a physician before undertaking any of the
advice, massage sequences, or using any of the products
suggested in this book. While every attempt has been
made to ensure the information in this book is correct and
up to date at the time of publication, the publisher accepts
no responsibility for consequences of the advice herein. If
in any doubt as to the nature of your condition, consult a
qualified medical practitioner.

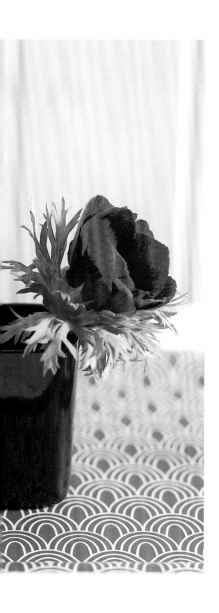

contents

introduction

This book is the evolution of my years of study, practice, and experience. I have modified the professional techniques I use to show you how to give a simple, yet profound, healing massage to friends, family, and yourself.

While it is not intended to be a substitute for professional help, this book introduces the philosophies and healing techniques of the East and West that have informed my treatment style and inspired my own journey of self-discovery. From my travels in China and training in South East Asia to nearly 20 years of practice in London and Vancouver, where I now live, I bring you an authentic fusion of the East and West to relax, heal, and replenish mind and body.

We all have a natural ability to promote healing in ourselves and others. Whether you're a curious beginner or someone who is contemplating training as a professional, reading these pages will empower you to find your own unique pathway into massage and healing. Within this book, you'll find easy-to-integrate techniques of massage, healing, meditation, aromatherapy, acupressure, Traditional Chinese Medicine (TCM), Ayurvedic massage, and reflexology. As you progress, you'll steadily be able to develop the skills and knowledge you need to give a simple yet effective healing massage.

I have intentionally kept the techniques simple and repeated a few of them in different sequences to aid familiarity and ease of application. Where relevant, I've also added arrows to the massage sequence photographs, so you can see what to do at a glance.

how to use this book

Chapter 1: Massage Pure and Simple presents the basic techniques, a step-by-step, full-body massage, and a reflex foot massage.

In Chapter 2, I take you through energetic healing for yourself and others, working with the chakra energy centers, visualization, and an auric shower meditation for relaxation and renewal.

Chapter 3 travels to India to discover the ancient therapy of Ayurveda. In this section, you'll learn how to assess your "doshic" type, give an Ayurvedic massage or "Abhyanga," and use essential oil blends to balance your dosha.

Chapter 4: Acupressure explores Traditional Chinese Medicine, as I explain how to use acupressure to treat minor ailments and boost vitality. You can add acupressure to any of your massage treatments (however, do see the cautions for acupressure on pages 92 and 101). You'll notice how, for your ease, white dots clearly show the location of every point.

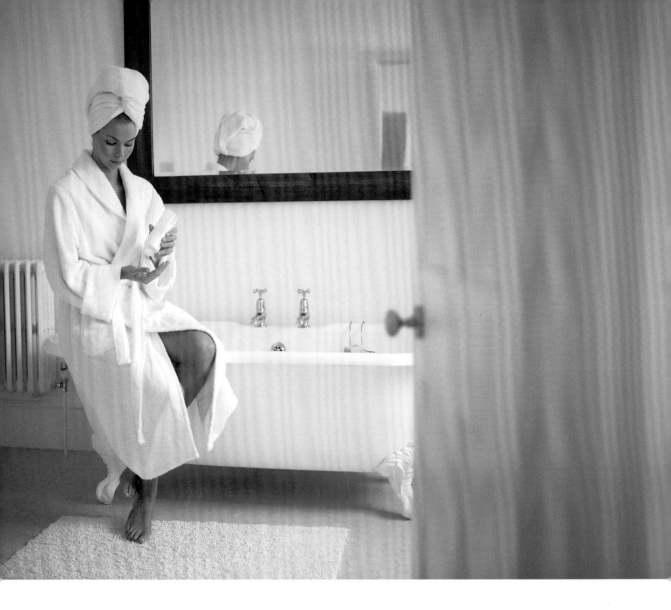

Massage on the Move, in Chapter 5, describes a unique massage program that I have developed for the busy world we live in today, featuring self-massage and massage for others on the move.

Chapter 6 explores nine essential oil profiles, to help you build the perfect aromatherapy kit, while Chapter 7 provides many health tips for various ailments, from headaches and common colds to fertility support.

I now invite you to begin your own journey into the world of healing and massage, and experience its relieving, uplifting, empowering, and life-changing effects for yourself.

Namaste,

Daphne Roubini

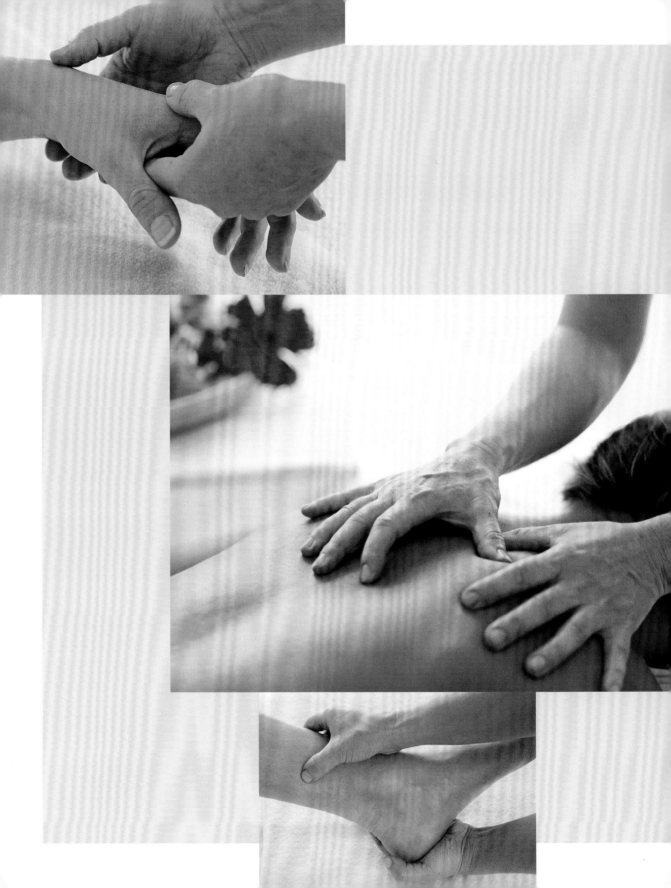

massage pure and simple

The pleasure of touch is a primal need. So little wonder that massage is one of the most profound ways of nurturing, soothing, and comforting a human being.

My earliest memory is being massaged with warm olive oil by my mother when I was a baby; I am now a qualified baby massage teacher, and it gives me great pleasure to see how much babies love to be massaged. I believe that the need to be touched does not diminish as we get older.

This chapter provides a foundation for all the massage sequences shown in this book. These basic steps are easy to follow, ideal for friends and family, and will make you feel like a comforted baby again.

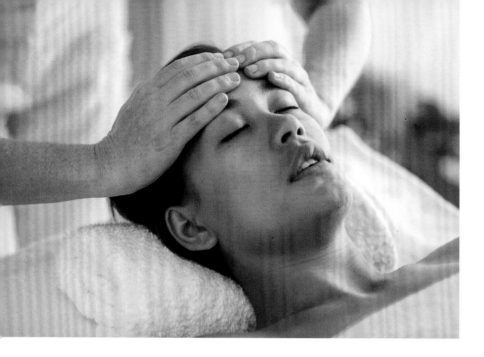

simple healing massage

This simple massage technique offers a simple yet powerful way to relieve the mild aches, strains, and muscle tension that can build up in our busy modern lives.

You can do this sequence on its own or include other techniques that I describe—a kind of a mix and match. For example, add an aromatic blend, or healing crystals, or include acupressure, or a guided cleansing visualization and your treatment becomes highly individual, tailored to your needs, and those of the recipient, at that moment.

This pure and simple massage is perfect for easing the normal stresses and strains of everyday life. But it is not designed to treat more serious health problems. If you have chronic back or joint pain, it is important that you seek treatment from a specialist medical practitioner before receiving a massage.

simple massage techniques

I have chosen the following techniques from my repertoire because they are easy to follow and perform, as well as being powerful, yet soothing tools for massage. As you massage, check that the pressure is at an enjoyable level. Massage should not be painful. I treat the recipient "layer by layer," with a constantly monitoring touch. Only then may I venture further by applying pressure that is a little deeper.

Before you start, check that the recipient is warm, comfortable, and does not feel over-exposed. If they are more comfortable wearing underwear, then that's perfectly okay. Use a sheet with a blanket and towels to cover any areas of the body that are not being massaged. Keep the recipient as cozy as possible and place a pillow under their ankles when they are lying on their tummy, and under their knees when they are lying on their back.

1 Applying the oil

Try to make the application of oil an enjoyable experience and as much a part of the massage as possible. Rest the nozzle of the bottle between your second and third finger, with your palm flat on the skin. Then apply the warmed oil as you move your hand in a seamless stroke. Alternatively, keep a little bowl of oil by your side and dip your fingers into the bowl and apply. The recipient is hypersensitive to your touch, so put all your attention into each move and make this initial contact really count, setting the tone for the rest of the massage.

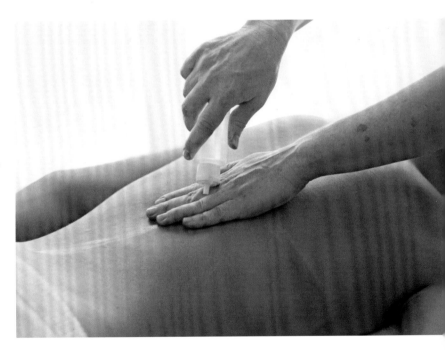

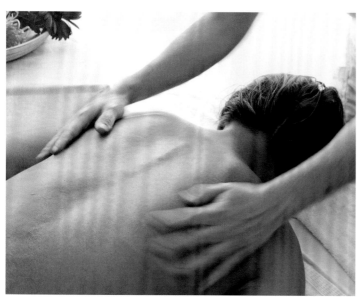

2 Long strokes

Massage manuals often call long strokes "effleurage," but I aim to keep the terminology as simple as I can—so long strokes it is. Keep your palms flat as you glide your hands up and down the body. You can either alternate your hands—right then left—or keep them side by side. Long strokes are best for large areas of the body, such as the back, and front and back of the legs. This is an excellent move to be repeated according to your intuition. It helps to flush toxins out of the muscles, and it feels great.

3 Kneading

Kneading is a standard massage stroke and can be used on the neck, legs, arms, and shoulders to ease tense muscles. Gently knead the flesh with rhythmic, slow, left-and-right motions, as if you are kneading dough.

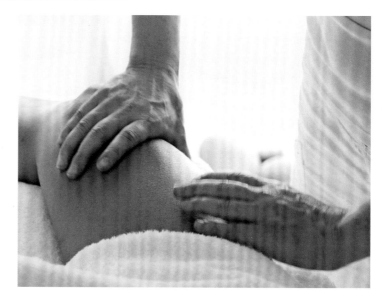

GETTING THE PRESSURE RIGHT

The recipient may be reticent to tell you if you are pressing too hard (even if you ask) so always look for signs of discomfort. Check to see if their face appears relaxed. See if the hands or feet are moving. Watch for wincing—an obvious sign of discomfort!

Then adjust the pressure. I find that using a deliberate but light touch melts the muscles more effectively than deep prodding.

4 Thumb rolling

Use a little pressure here to roll your thumbs into the muscles. Keep your thumbs close as you alternately roll them around each other. Thumb rolling is perfect for releasing any muscle knots you find as you massage, especially in the upper and lower back and hip area.

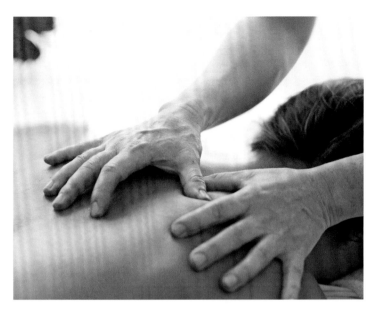

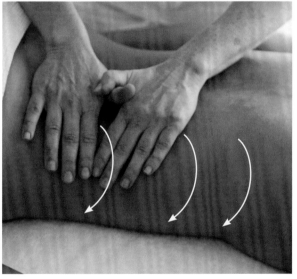

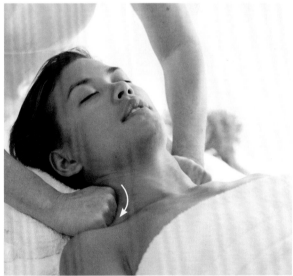

5 Butterfly hands

Connect both hands by linking the thumbs in a butterfly shape. This locks the hands together as you massage in circular motions around the sides of the body. This stroke can also be used to sweep down the sides of the spine, adding more strength and control.

6 Light fist rolling

Hold both hands in a fist shape and gently roll them into the neck and shoulders, to release any build-up of tension in the neck muscles. This stroke can also be used in the buttock area to release tension that can accumulate in the lower back and hip area (see page 99).

the back of the body

I like to begin a massage by working on the back, as most recipients cannot wait to have this part of their body treated. The little knots that you may find are due to lactic acid build-up in the muscle fibers.

Start with a rocking movement, which helps the recipient let go and really relax. This is a technique I learned as part of the Linn Transcadence massage, based on the tradition of the Native American Cherokee tribe.

Which side you work from depends on whether you are right- or left-handed. I'm right-handed, so I tend to favor the left side of my clients. If you're left-handed, swap the directions that I describe from right to left.

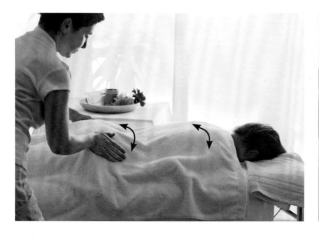

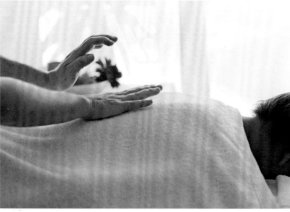

1 With the recipient on their front, covered by a towel, start by just making contact. Be present in your intention and confidence (see box, opposite). Place your left hand on the upper back, where shoulders and neck meet, and your right hand on the base of the spine (not shown). Now rock back and forth gently. This makes the connection between you and the recipient as well as gently rocking away the tension stored in the muscles, spine, and joints. We were all babies once and I often think how good it must have felt to be soothed by being rocked. Rock gently seven times. Next, put both hands gently and unobtrusively onto both hips (left) and rock back and forth. This releases the tension in the hip and legs. Rock for three sets of seven.

2 With the recipient's back still covered, walk your palms up the back, applying pressure to the sides of the spine as you go. This step is called "cat padding." It connects you with the recipient and helps them to begin to slow down and releases tension in the back.

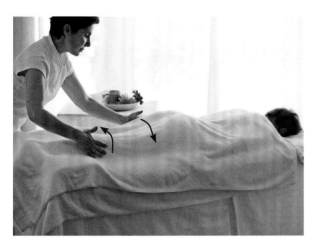

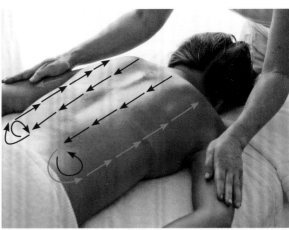

3 Rock the hips again, this time including the legs. Then sweep your hands down the back of the legs, rocking as you go. Finish with both palms resting on the soles of the feet. This relaxes and integrates the whole body, giving a wonderful sense of freedom and connection.

4 Uncover the back and apply the oil using a flat palm down the center of the spine, as shown in technique 1 (see page 11). Then follow the arrows in this picture for application of the oil over the rest of the back. Now sweep your hands down the back, on either side of the spine, and across the waist. Circle into the waist and tops of the hips, then continue back up and over the shoulders and down the arms. This move really builds on the relaxing experience of the massage.

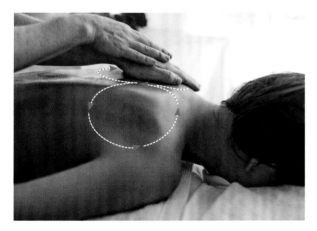

5 At the side of the recipient now, place one hand on top of the other and apply deeper pressure as you stroke around the shoulders and the top of the back in a figure of eight. This step releases the trapezium muscle and is perfect for tired or aching shoulders. This technique is repeated later in step 12 around the hips, the perfect way to easily apply more pressure that remains both enjoyable and effective.

MAKING CONTACT

Always be present in your intention and confidence as you massage—stay focused on your contact with the recipient and concentrate on the strokes you are giving. Always bear in mind that the person is in a heightened mode of sensitivity and is acutely aware of your every move. They will easily pick up on a sense of detachment, for example, if your mind starts to wander. For truly healing massage it is important to put your own concerns and worries to one side and make contact with the recipient on every level—not just physical but mental, emotional, and spiritual as well.

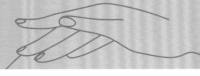

6 Knead the neck gently with cupped hands. The right hand follows the contour of the neck from the top of the shoulder to the point where it meets the base of the skull. The left hand repeats this movement going the other way. This is a blissful way to relax the neck. Stay doing this for a while. It is always greatly appreciated. Now repeat step 5 and this step for three or four rounds.

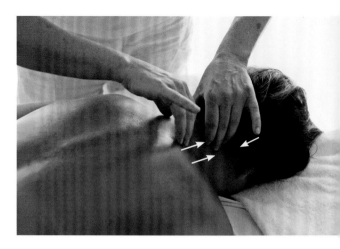

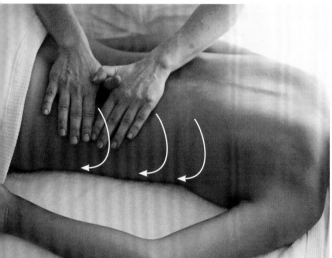

7 Use "butterfly hands" to massage the body in circular strokes, first on the right side of the body and then on the left side. This step helps to relieve tension and also enhances our breathing. This is because it aids healthy respiration, helping the body to get adequate oxygen. Now switch sides and repeat the "butterfly hands" stroke.

8 Standing or kneeling at the recipient's head, sweep your hands down the back, creating a double figure of eight that completes with a sweep down both arms. Do this in a set of seven. This step can also be performed from the side of the recipient, beginning at the hips and moving upwards. Repeat this movement at any time in the massage.

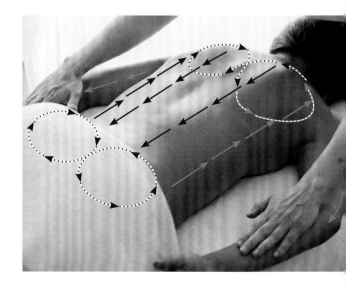

9 Still at the head of the recipient, roll your thumbs around the upper back to work out any knots you find in the trapezium muscle. This step eases stiff shoulders and neck, and relieves tension headaches. It is so enjoyable for the recipient you may want to repeat this section as many times as feels comfortable (trust your instinct). Ask the recipient to let you know if there is any discomfort at all. If so, adjust the pressure.

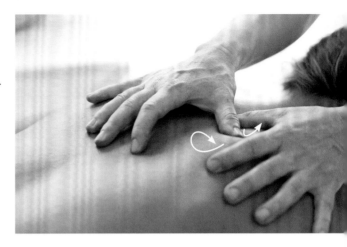

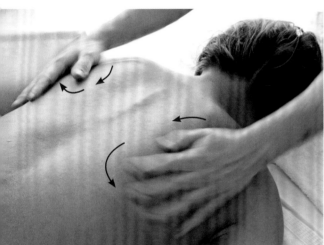

10 Continue with double-handed circular sweeps around the shoulder blades. This step softens the muscles here and helps boost the blood circulation and lymphatic system. Return to the side of the recipient and rock the hips. This releases the whole back even further. One of my clients describes this rocking movement as "feeling as if my back muscles are melting off my spine."

11 Massage the sacrum by rolling your thumbs into any tense areas. This is particularly useful to relieve lower back ache if you have been driving or sitting a lot, or suffering menstrual cramps.

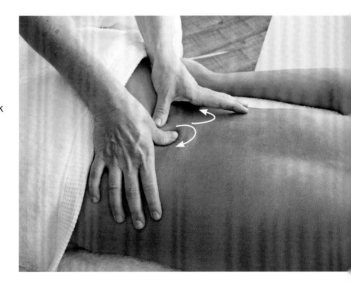

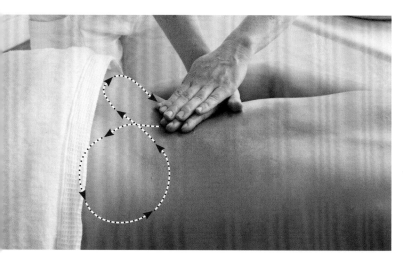

12 Massage the lower back by placing one hand on top of the other and making a figure of eight over hips and lower back. This is an effective way to relieve lower backache. Spend time here.

13 Use your hands with flat palms to "cat pad" up the back, one hand following the other like the steps of a slow, stealthy cat. Use some pressure here. This is another very simple technique you can use to release tension in the back.

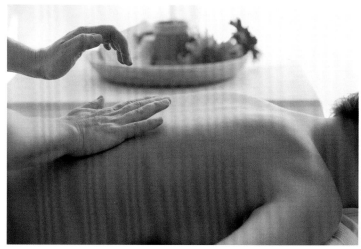

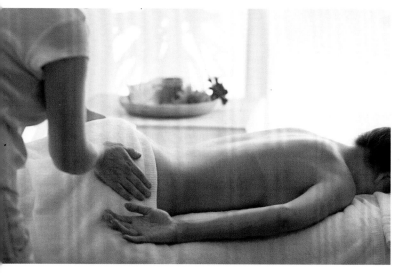

14 Do another set of rocking to complete this back massage. Cover the recipient and complete by holding one hand on the upper back and one on the lower back for a while. Now lift off your hands very gently, imagining that their soothing quality remains behind.

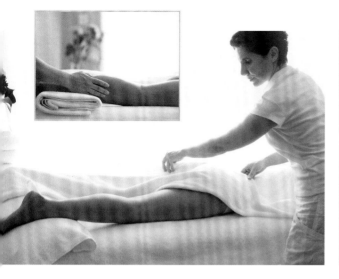

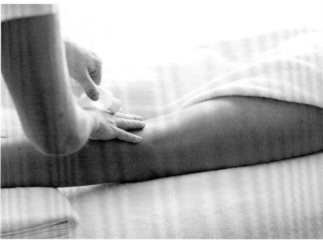

15 Make sure the recipient is comfortable by adjusting the pillow. Holding the ankles in your two hands, lift up both legs and swing them gently. Then drape the towel discreetly over the other leg.

16 Apply oil along the midline of the leg (remember to make this an enjoyable part of the massage). This helps to unwind the calf muscle. This step is one of my personal favorites.

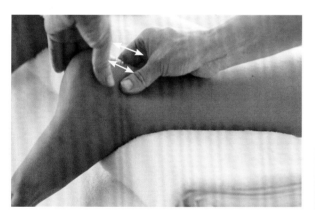

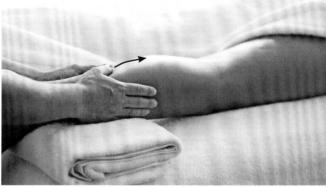

17 Using your thumbs and first fingers, gently knead the Achilles tendon. This is a relieving point for the whole leg and foot and releases any tension that can build up after a day spent on your feet.

18 With thumbs placed side by side, trace the center of the calf. This step eases the gastrocnemius muscle and, again, releases tension caused by walking a lot—especially when wearing high heels.

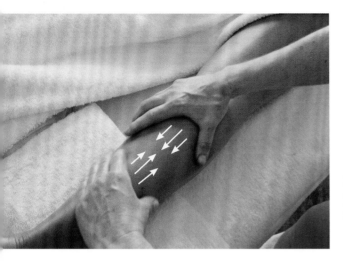

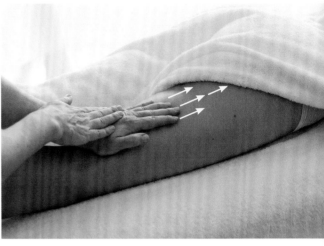

19 Holding both hands in cup shapes, knead the whole calf muscle with a right to left motion. This step helps boost the blood circulation and releases tension in the lower leg.

20 Place your hands flat, with one hand on top of the other hand, and use some pressure to push up along the back of the thigh. This step aids the blood circulation and lymphatic drainage in the upper thigh.

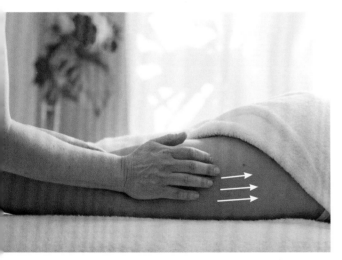

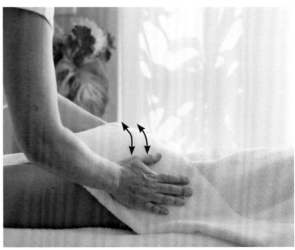

21 Use the heels of your hand to lightly sweep up the sides of the thighs. This movement is another good manual lymph-drainage technique and is especially useful if congestion or cellulite is present.

22 Use both hands to push and rock the hips and sacrum. This step helps release the hips and boosts the blood circulation in the whole lower leg area, as well as being very relaxing generally.

23 Interleave your fingers and sweep your hands over the whole leg, allowing them to separate and retrace lightly as they go back to the ankle. Repeat this seven times. This step completes the leg massage.

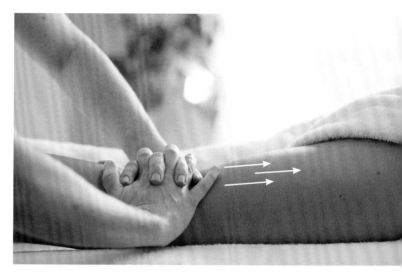

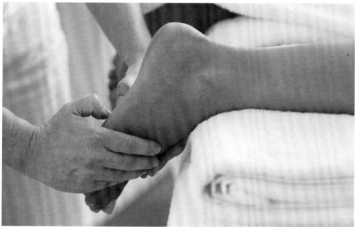

24 Now roll your thumbs over the sole of the foot. This is a great foot-tension reliever, useful for those with fallen arches, or who spend much of the day on their feet; it helps you let go and relax.

25 Holding the foot with one hand, push and sweep the palm of the other down the sole of the foot. Repeat this three times. End by holding the foot to ground the energy. Repeat on the other leg.

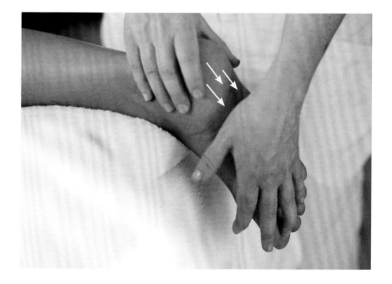

neck and face

Tension can build up in our face as we often have to put on a brave face or hide our true feelings. I find that people really appreciate having a facial massage; it is a real stress relief and deeply enhances a relaxed, radiant, and youthful glow.

Only a small amount of oil is needed here. This is a special part of the massage, so be light and very focused as people are rarely touched on their face and will be aware of your every move.

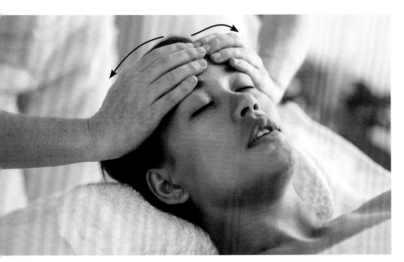

1 Place your fingertips at the midline of the forehead and stroke outward. This step quickly releases tension stored in the forehead from over-concentrating, and can ease headaches and tiredness.

2 With your thumb and first finger, gently pinch along the brow line at each dot position. This is perfect for relieving headaches and eyestrain—blissful after a long day sitting at the computer.

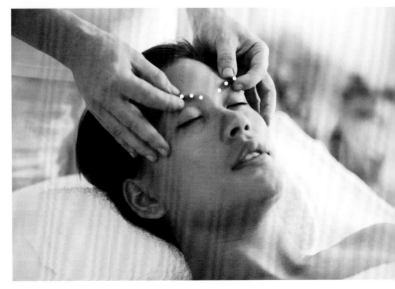

3 With your first finger, gently press all around the orbital bone as shown (taking great care not to work too close to the eyeball!). This step is great for easing tension headaches caused by close-up work involving the eyes and for general eye strain.

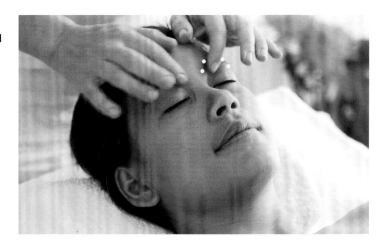

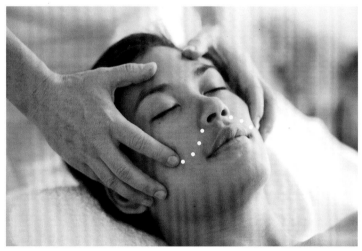

4 With palms resting against the sides of the head, use your first fingers simultaneously to trace the lines of the sinuses underneath the cheekbones, pressing at each dot as shown. This is a great way to relieve blocked sinuses due to hay fever, sinusitis, colds, or flu.

5 Using both hands, cup the jaw and massage using sweeping outward movements. This is an easy way to release jaw tension, especially in those who "swallow their anger" or grind their teeth.

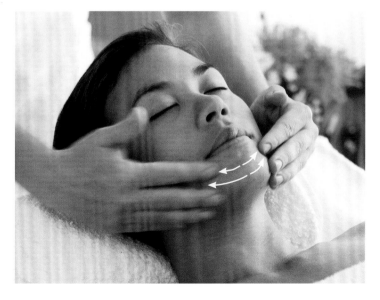

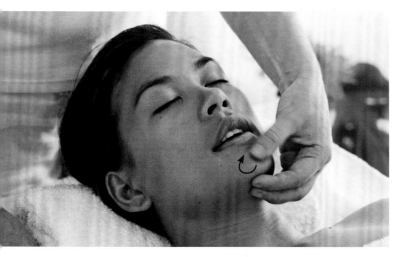

6 Use a rotating "thumb roll" movement to circle the chin area. This relieves jaw tension and feels great. We all hold a lot of tension in our faces from putting on a brave face. Try using both thumbs here.

7 Again using your thumbs, make circular movements around the forehead. This is good for smoothing furrows and tension lines, enhancing a real sense of freedom all over the head.

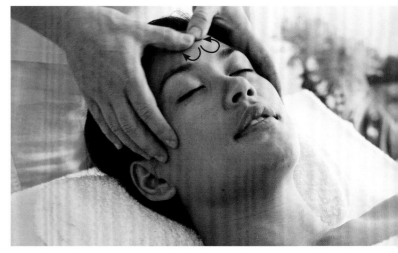

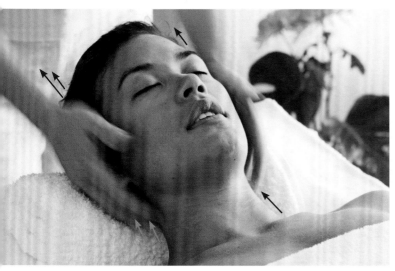

8 Starting at the back of the neck, use your hands to make a sweeping motion that stretches the back of the neck. Complete this move by sweeping your fingers through the hair three times.

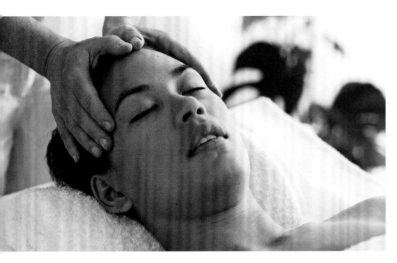

9 Place your palms on top of the head and hold, gently resting your hands in position. Visualize bright light and healing sunshine filling the recipient from head to toe. Unusual if you haven't tried healing yet but you will soon get it. Do this for 1–3 minutes, or as long as you like.

10 Now "cat pad" on the shoulders with both hands alternately, right and then left. This feels very calming and helps release tension in the neck and shoulders.

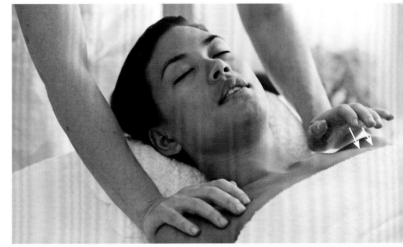

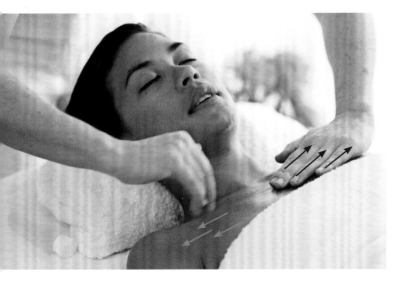

11 Apply more oil using alternating sweeping strokes across chest. This step relaxes the upper chest muscles and eases constricted breathing.

12 Make your hands into fists and roll them gently into the tops of the shoulders. Gradually build up the pressure here as you get more confident and the recipient gives you feedback on how much pressure they like.

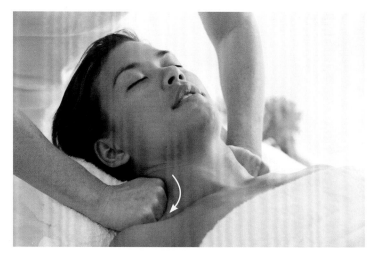

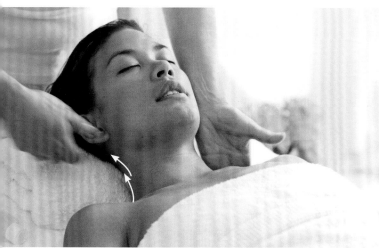

13 Use sweeping movements, right to left, along the back of the neck (think of gently pulling a rope, hand under hand) and always be careful and rhythmic. Repeat step 10 ("cat padding") along the shoulders and then repeat step 9, holding the head and channeling light as this releases and settles any accumulated energy.

14 Using both hands as shown, turn the head to the side and allow the face to rest in your left hand on the pillow. This movement prepares for the next step.

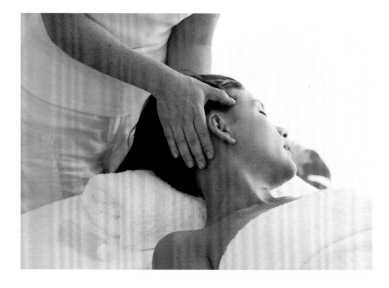

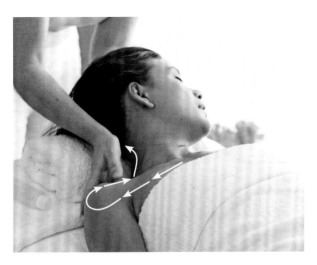

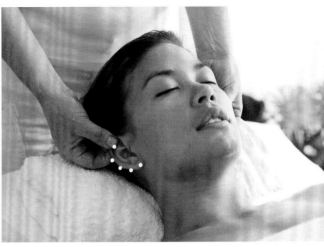

15 Still gently supporting the head with one hand, sweep the other hand across the front of the top of the chest, from the midline, around the shoulder to the upper back and neck seven times. Repeat on the other side. Repeat this step, and step 12 (fist rolling).

16 Massage both ears simultaneously by gently pressing them between your thumbs and first fingers. Repeat three times. In acupuncture and auricular reflexology, massaging the ears can benefit all parts of the recipient and is more relaxing than you might imagine.

CAUTION

Take care to avoid working the front of the neck. Always keep behind the muscles of the sternocleidomastoid, the large muscle at the side of the neck.

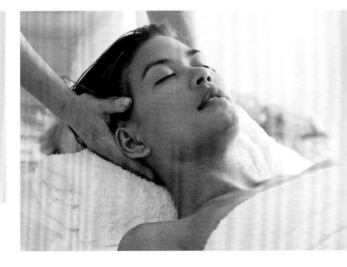

17 Using both hands and keeping your fingers soft, gently support and hold the occipital ridges (natural bumps and dents) in the skull. Let the head rest here for a while. This induces a deep sense of relaxation and helps release tension along the spine.

arms and hands

We do so much repetitive work with our hands and arms, it is little wonder we often feel tense and achy at the end of the day. The steps described here are perfect for relieving any build-up of tension that may occur, for example, due to driving or computer work.

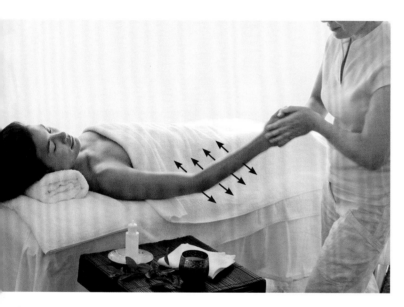

1 Hold the recipient's hand with both of yours—your right palm against their left palm, as shown. Pull the arm out to shoulder level and shake it out. This releases initial tension in the arm and shoulder.

2 Apply the massage oil using sweeping movements along the whole arm, up and around the back of the shoulder, and back down to the hand again.

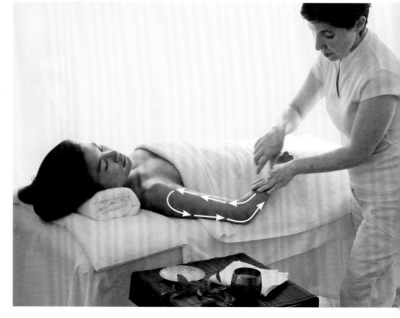

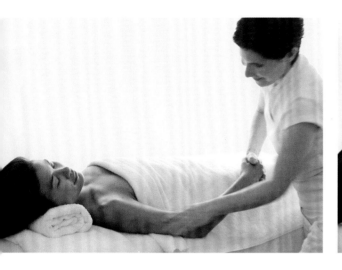

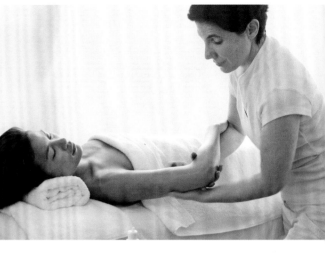

3 Hold the wrist with your right hand and massage the arm with your left hand using long sweeping strokes. This stimulates the circulation and eases muscle tension, especially the kind that builds up due to prolonged computer use, driving or other repetitive movement.

4 Lift the arm up, holding the elbow in your right hand and resting their forearm on your right inner forearm. Now sweep behind the upper arm with your left hand. This massages the triceps, an often-neglected muscle group, and feels so relaxing.

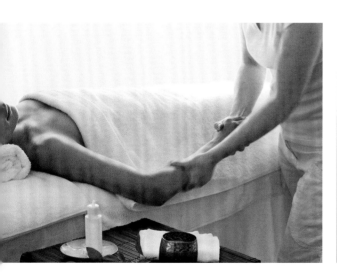

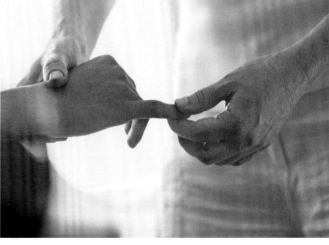

5 Hold the recipient's hand with your right hand and sweep up the forearm with your cupped left hand. This step releases more tension in the forearm, as well as boosting the circulation in the arm.

6 Gently shake out, massage, and squeeze each finger, working on each joint as well as the whole finger. Begin with the little finger and then work through each finger in turn. Finish with the thumb.

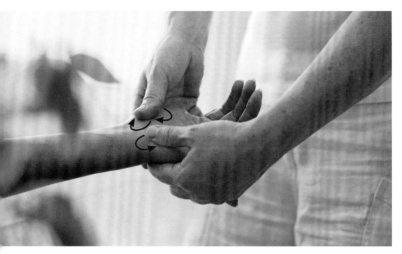

7 Turn the hand upwards and interlink your little fingers between their little finger and third finger, and their first finger and thumb. Then "thumb roll" the recipient's palm. This releases any tension held in the hand.

8 Hold the recipient's hand with your left hand and massage into the channels of the forearm with your right thumb, working the left, middle, and right channel as shown. Repeat step 1 (shake out the arm) and step 3 (long stroke over the front of the arm).

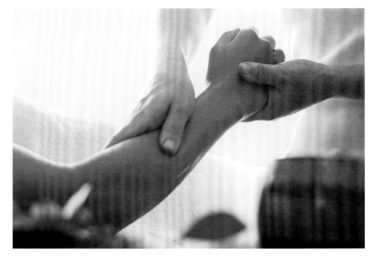

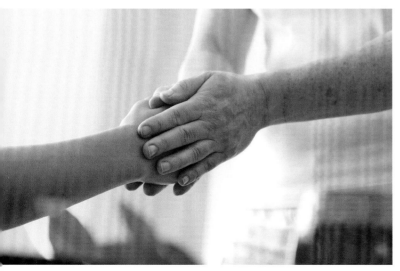

9 Hold the recipient's hand between both of your palms. This step feels very comforting. It stills the energy you have been moving around and completes the sequence on this arm. Repeat on the other arm.

front of legs

This sequence focuses on the legs and feet, relieving aching and tension caused by exercise, or the result of long periods spent on your feet or sitting at a desk.

1 Hold the ankle confidently and raise the leg, gently swinging it from left to right. Now gently place it on the massage table with a pillow under the knee. This helps release the hips and puts the recipient in a comfortable position. Repeat on the other leg, then hold and lift both legs, and swing them gently to further release the hips.

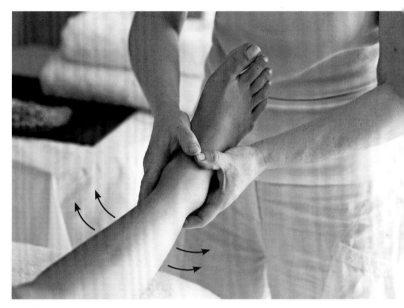

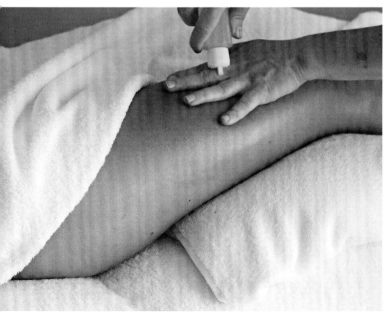

2 Apply the oil with long sweeps up to the knee and then up over the front of the thigh (not forgetting to make this part of the massage as enjoyable as possible!). Maintain the relaxed energy you have already created.

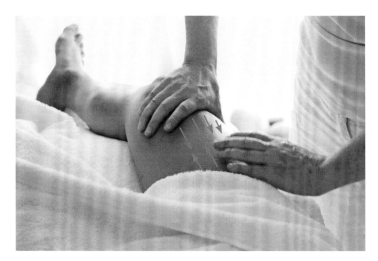

3 Use both hands to knead the front of the upper thigh. This releases the thigh muscle and eases any tension that may have accumulated, for example, due to excessive cycling, stair climbing, or gym work.

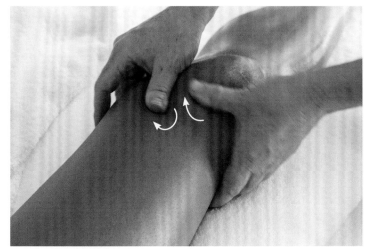

4 Gently "thumb roll" around the kneecap. Be careful here as the knees are very delicate joints so do not press on the kneecap itself. This simple move can be very relieving if there is tension or aching due to, for example, prolonged sitting or driving.

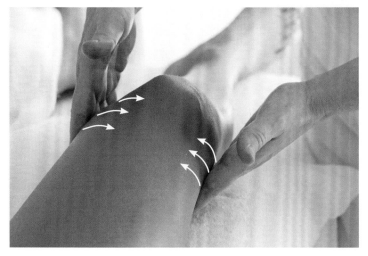

5 Sweep your hands up gently from behind the knee. Again, be careful here as the knees are very delicate. This simple move can be very relieving if there is any tension in the knees or legs, for example, as a result of sitting at a desk for hours.

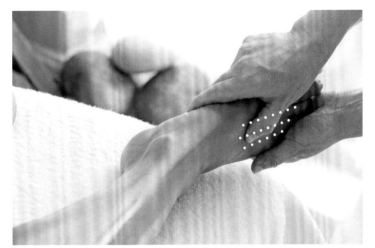

6 Gently use your thumbs to trace the grooves on the top of the foot that mark the spaces between the foot bones. This move releases the tension in the whole foot and also stimulates the reflexology points for the chest and diaphragm.

7 Now apply double-handed sweeps over the whole leg, ending with the feet. This move connects the leg with the foot. To aid the circulation, use more pressure on the way up and a lighter touch on the way down so that you are massaging the blood towards the heart.

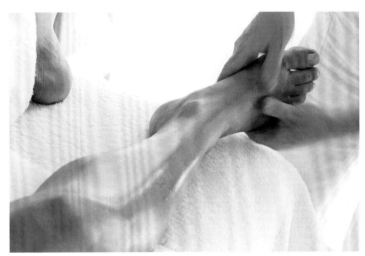

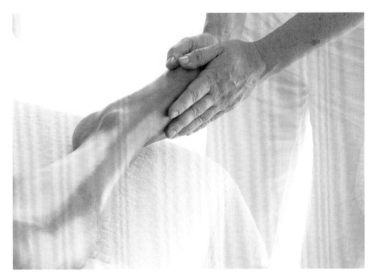

8 Use both hands to hold the recipient's foot like a slipper. This move settles the energy of the leg as well as helping to make the person feel grounded, centered, and secure in the world. If you want to extend the foot massage, follow the sequence on pages 37–39 to complete this simple healing massage.

reflex foot massage

Although reflexology has only become well known in the West relatively recently, it is by no means a new form of therapy. Pressure point massage of the feet was practiced by the ancient Egyptians, early Chinese, North American Indian tribes, and 16th-century European physicians.

Reflexology is based on the principle that every organ and working system within the body has a mirror reflex point located in the foot, and that by massaging these points it is possible to detect and treat illness, improve levels of health, and give a general feeling of wellbeing.

I have incorporated some of the foot reflex points of the Rwo-shur Health method, a form of reflexology I studied in Malaysia, and based this reflex foot massage sequence on the various massage techniques I know to give you an introduction to reflexology as well as an amazing healing sequence that is much more than just a foot rub.

getting started

I did my reflexology apprenticeship at Peter Lim's clinic in Melaka, Malaysia. Here, clients were seated side by side while we sat on low stools with the patient's foot resting on little towels on our laps. Everyone was noisily chatting to each other—not the peaceful Zen environment Western visitors often expect and respond to—but the effects of the treatment were still astonishing!

Make sure the recipient is sitting comfortably, or lying on a bed, with you seated close by on a lower stool, and rest their foot on a clean hand towel in your lap. I like to use a small sushi bowl for massage oil. Unlike bottles, it is easy to access and unlikely to fall over. Place the dish within easy reach. Always keep one hand on the recipient, and use the other to reach and administer the oil. In this way you can maintain the momentum of the massage without needing to take your hands away each time you have to apply more oil. See the aromatherapy chapter (pages 130–135) for suggestions for essential oil blends to use here. I love reflexology and recommend it as a potent aid to general health and relaxation.

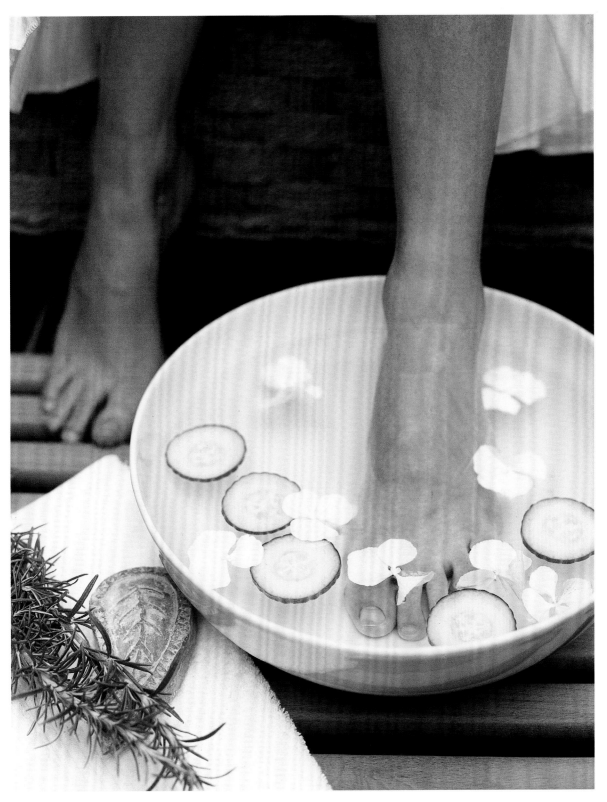

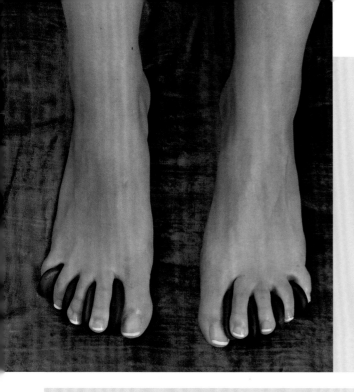

SEA-STONE BLISS

Reflex zone therapy is a branch of reflexology that divides the body into perpendicular zones that run throughout the body.

Little stones can be placed between the toes to open the reflex zones in the feet. This clears the energetic pathways throughout the body. I harvested my sea stones on one of the Northern Gulf Islands, off Vancouver Island, Canada. Next time you are on a beach, look for eight smooth stones to fit between your toes. I believe that stones absorb the energies of minerals, earth, sun, and sea, and add an extra dimension to any healing treatment.

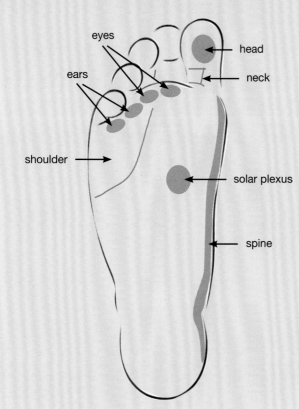

SOLE BENEFITS

This reflex foot massage is designed to activate reflex points on the soles of the feet to release any tension in the following areas of the body: the head and neck, eyes and ears, shoulder, spine, and solar plexus. A visit to a professional reflexologist will enable you to experience the complete treatment.

regenerating reflex foot massage

This is a potent foot massage sequence that can be used on its own or in combination with the simple healing massage (see page 10).

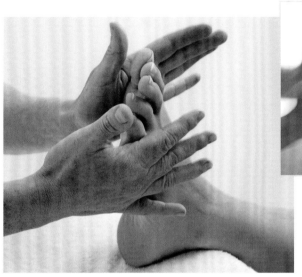

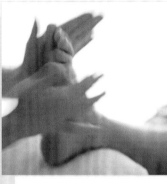

1 Begin by holding the left foot between your parallel hands and roll it between your right and left hand, shaking the foot out.

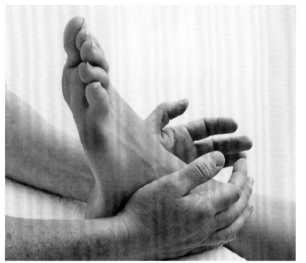

2 Use the heels of your palms in a rapid movement alternating from right to left to release the ankle.

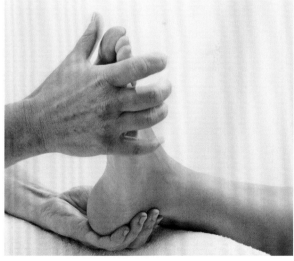

3 Holding the ankle with your left hand, rotate the foot with your right hand—first to your right and then to your left.

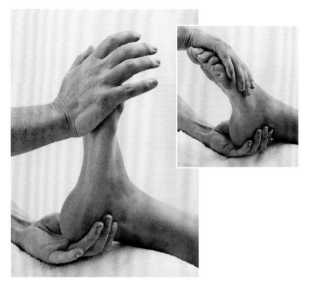

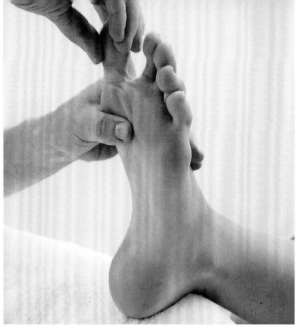

4 Continuing to hold the ankle with your left hand, gently flex and extend the foot with your right hand.

5 Gently pull, bend, and then rotate each toe, starting with the little toe—this stimulates the eye and ear points. Spend longer rotating the big toes in both directions at least eight times, as this can really help to release the neck area.

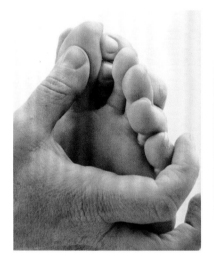

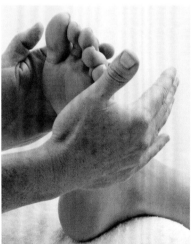

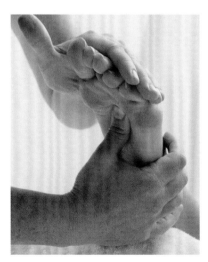

6 Work the pad of the big toe with your right thumb while supporting the back of the toe with your left. This stimulates the head points and releases tension in the head.

7 Roll the foot between both palms and then roll the ankle again. Spend some time continuing to shake the foot out.

8 Hold your right thumb over the solar plexus point and gently pull the foot over the point using your left hand. This calms the mind and nerves.

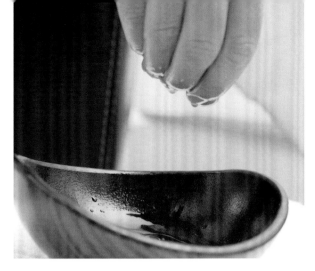

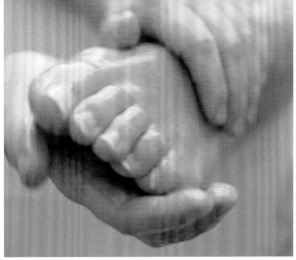

9 Administer oil—dip your fingertips into the oil and build up "the slip" each time. The foot needs to be lightly lubricated so that your hand slips easily, but not so slippery that you can't apply any pressure. Try to make the application of oil a soothing, enjoyable experience for the recipient, rather than an interruption in the session.

10 Massage the foot with smooth, long strokes. Aim to build a lovely rhythmic sense here. Count sets of five strokes. Do this at least 15 times.

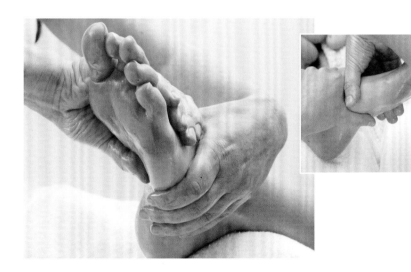

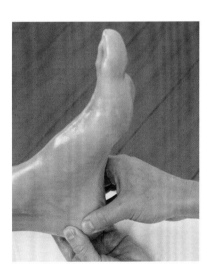

11 Use a gentle rhythmic wringing movement along the instep. This releases the spine reflex points and feels wonderful. Repeat this for a while. Alternate between steps 10 and 11 to really build up a deep sense of relaxation.

12 Use a thumb-rolling movement around the area where the base of the foot meets the heel—this helps to affect the releasing of the coccyx and sacrum. Complete this foot massage by holding the foot between both your hands and imagining golden light pouring out of your hands, calming and grounding the recipient.

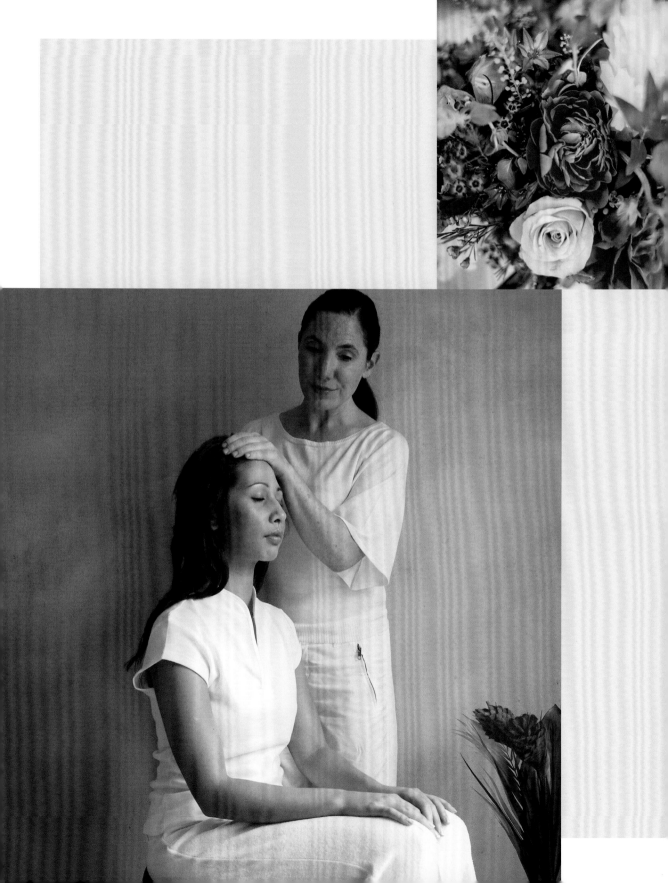

energetic healing and visualization

Throughout history and in all the world's cultures there have been people who had the gift of healing. Sometimes this gift was nurtured within a religious community, such as Buddhist monks. At other times the person with the gift was simply the village healer or soothsayer.

In the past, the ability to heal could arouse suspicion and even fear—of witchcraft, of the unknown, of the rationally inexplicable. Yet healing is natural, easy, and can be nurtured within us all to use for ourselves and for friends, partners, and family.

This next sequence is simple to follow and provides an introduction to the fascinating world of energetic healing. It has been derived from a wide range of Eastern and Western healing traditions and forms an ideal starting point for those who wish to try this approach to touch therapy.

The sequence starts with meditation and visualization techniques to help you prepare for giving healing. It is the ideal way to begin your own journey of self-healing and can become part of the dynamic that defines your own world.

visualization

Visualization is a powerful aid to healing. The brain does not differentiate between what is real and what is perceived, either in the imagination or memory.

We all know how thinking about a bad experience from our past makes us cringe as if it was all happening over again. Similarly, if you remember a happy experience, for example the sun on your face as you sit with your dog on the beach, you will feel as if you are actually there. We can use this knowledge to heal ourselves and others. Next time you feel caught up in a sad past experience, try this "switching" technique: think of a very happy past experience in great detail, then switch the memories.

Imagination is part of how we create. Creation begins in thought and then becomes matter. Visualization is nothing more than a refined form of imagination. Visualizing or imagining healing yourself or others is actually a natural, unconscious part of our everyday lives. You can harness this natural ability for your highest good.

As part of the preparation for giving a healing massage, I will explain how to connect with the body's energy centers, or chakras, which are an important part of the ancient Indian healing tradition of Ayurveda. On the following pages I describe the seven chakras, their locations in the body, and their physical, emotional, and spiritual properties. You can also use crystals to balance the chakras, if you wish, and I explain how to do this later in this section. You could choose a crystal in advance by consulting the information on the chakras on pages 44–48. This is not a necessity, however, as this contained healing sequence will promote a general sense of wellbeing, peace, and relaxation.

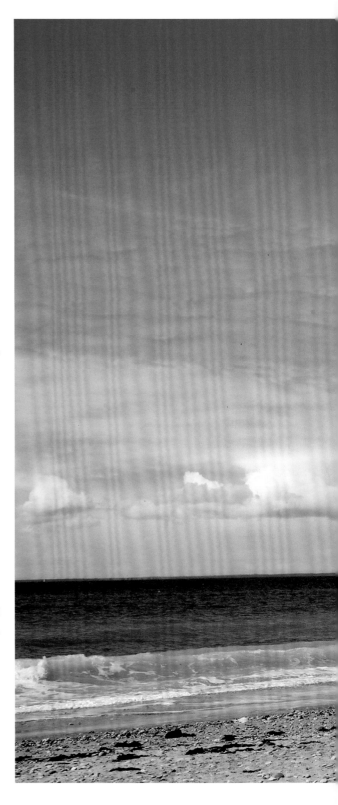

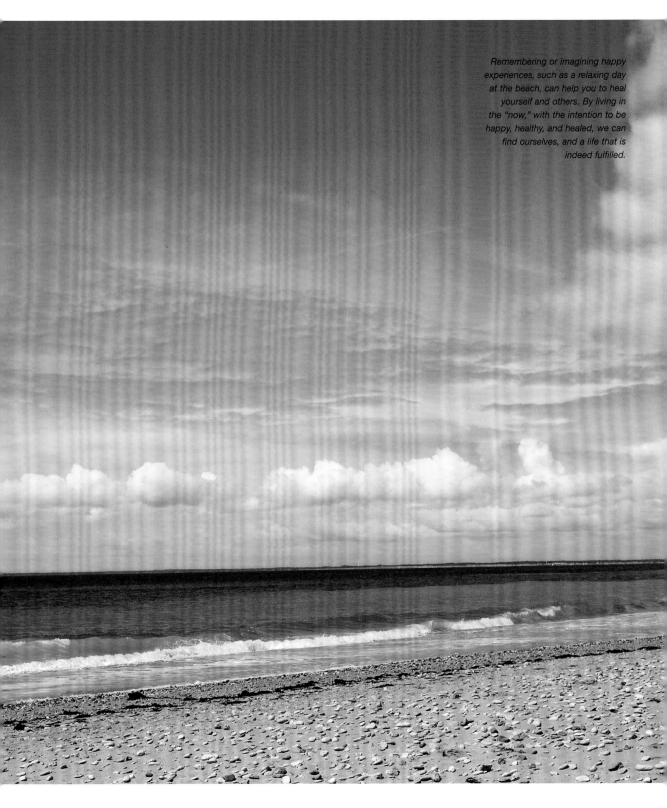

Remembering or imagining happy experiences, such as a relaxing day at the beach, can help you to heal yourself and others. By living in the "now," with the intention to be happy, healthy, and healed, we can find ourselves, and a life that is indeed fulfilled.

chakras

Chakras, or energy centers, are described throughout ancient Ayurvedic texts. This ancient concept comes from the Sanskrit word "chakrum," which means spinning wheel. A chakra can be described as a vortex of energy. It performs as an antennae that receives universal energy directly into the auric structure of the body. Chakras are the body's way of connecting with the universal energy that links us all. These energetic centers make us potent in the world in all our aspects—physically, mentally, emotionally, and spiritually. They help us feel truly vital and alive, enlivened by the world around us and by our authentic place in it.

Chakras are not visible, except to those gifted healers who have the ability to "see" the aura and the chakras with their inner vision, intuition, or psychic sensitivity. These healers can make interesting diagnoses based on the physical, emotional, or spiritual imbalances they "see" in the auric structure and may suggest solutions accordingly. These may be through an auric healing session, a visualized meditation, or a change of diet or thought structure. *Hands of Light* by Barbara Brennan (see page 144) has more information on this kind of healing session.

The notion of energy centers can be challenging to contemplate if the concept is new to you, but with openness of mind and some imagined visualization you too can have these powerhouses of vitality and spirit at your proverbial fingertips. For the moment, just use your imagination and intention to explore this fascinating way to see your own body. It is not necessary to see the aura to know that it is there or imagine being in touch with it. It will happen anyway, so don't be daunted. Give it a go. You don't have to see the bottom of the ocean to know it is there! I firmly believe that energy follows thought. Try it and see. It is no different from imagining sitting on a lovely beach or planning your evening meal while on the bus. And we all know how to do that!

I have listed the positions and characteristics of each chakra so that when you come to do the chakra visualization meditation or try some of the healing techniques, with or without crystals, you will have a good foundation to work from.

Look carefully at the physical region of each chakra, its life aspect, and how it may improve things for you when the chakra is truly in balance. For example, if you are experiencing a sore throat, this may be because your throat chakra is out of balance. Is there something you are holding back from saying? Something you need to say? Something you are sad about? Something you want to shout about? I have a friend who is a singer. She once lost her voice when her father died, and the sadness of that loss choked her voice for over two years. So, meditating on this chakra bringing light and energy to it, or using a lapis stone to raise the color vibration of the chakra may help heal the sore throat, sadness, grief, or the situation that needs communication.

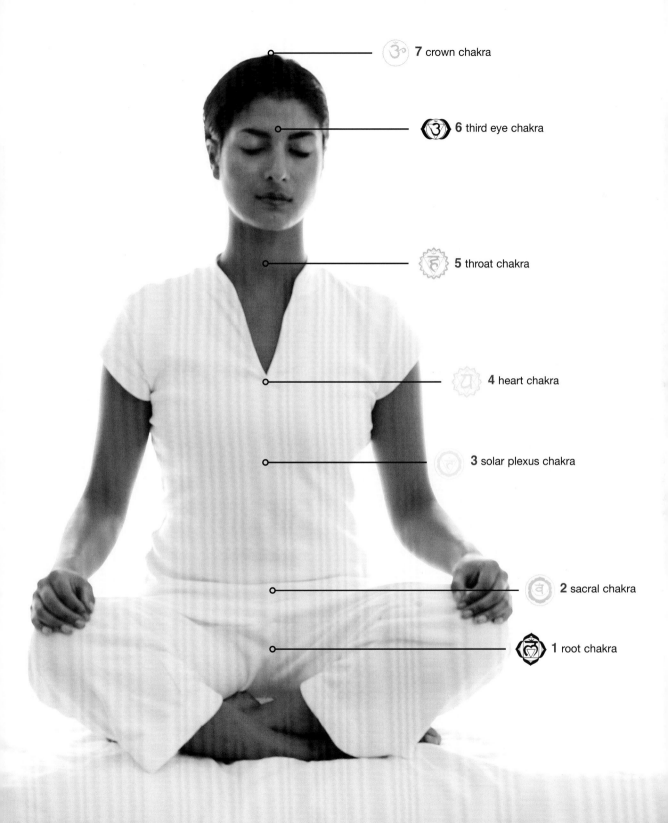

7 crown chakra

6 third eye chakra

5 throat chakra

4 heart chakra

3 solar plexus chakra

2 sacral chakra

1 root chakra

first chakra: root chakra

Sanskrit name: Muladhara
Position: At the root of the spine
Color: Red
Crystal: Ruby/agate
Endocrine gland: Adrenals
Physical region: Kidney, spine, and muscles
Life aspect: Grounded, stable, pertains to Earthly success, survival instinct, personal boundaries, and sexual power.

Cherry red Alaskan garnet

Root chakra in balance: Helps relieve a tendency to self-sabotage, or to hold ourselves back. This chakra helps us have a healthy sense of our physical needs such as rest and food. It is the seat of our physical power and in balance gives us a healthy, secure platform for balanced spiritual exploration.

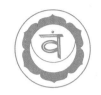

second chakra: sacral chakra

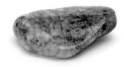

Sanskrit name: Svadhisthana
Position: Between the navel and genitals
Color: Orange
Crystal: Fire opal, carnelian
Endocrine gland: Genitals
Physical region: Reproductive organs, stomach, and colon
Life aspect: Sexuality, creativity, ability to enjoy life, and trust in yourself and others.

Orange moss agate

Sacral chakra in balance: Helps relieve sexual inhibition, and promotes fertility and a healthy libido. This chakra enhances one's ability to transform anger to understanding and wisdom. It is the chakra that helps us process life and let go of what we no longer need and keep what is still valuable to us. It is the chakra of creation and creativity.

third chakra: solar plexus chakra

Sanskrit name: Manipura
Position: Midway between the navel and ribcage
Color: Yellow
Crystal: Topaz, amber, citrine
Endocrine gland: Pancreas
Physical region: Stomach, liver and gall bladder, spleen, and nervous system

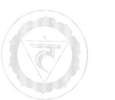

Smoky citrine

Life aspect: Instinct, will, humanity, personal power, a strong sense of self, and a continued sense of innocence.

Solar plexus chakra in balance: Helps us let go of fear and lack of self-esteem. Gives us a strong sense of who we are and what is right for us in the present. This chakra is our source of comfort, contentment, warmth, and security.

fourth chakra: heart chakra

Sanskrit name: Anahata
Position: The center of the breastbone or sternum
Color: Green
Crystal: Jade or malachite
Endocrine gland: Thymus gland
Physical region: Heart, blood, lower lungs, circulatory system, and diaphragm

Inca jade

Life aspect: Love, sympathy, community, peace, compassion, openness, ability to give and receive, and self-expression.

Heart chakra in balance: Helps us accept ourselves and others. It is the balance point for all other chakras governing our relationships and ability to relate to others. It helps us follow our authentic path in life and express genuine love.

fifth chakra: throat chakra

Sanskrit name: Vishuddha

Position: At the throat

Color: Blue

Crystal: Lapis lazuli

Endocrine gland: Thyroid

Physical region: Voice, upper lungs, and respiratory system

Life aspect: Allows us to communicate thoughts and feelings, release sadness, and directly relates to expressing inner creativity and empathy.

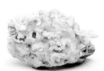

Lazulite

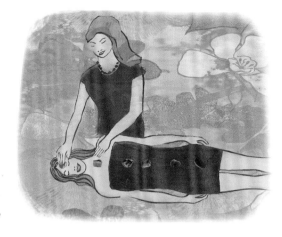

Throat chakra in balance: Helps release sadness, and promotes free confident creative expression, an ability to communicate with love and truth, and an ease of teaching and learning. Together with a balanced heart, the throat chakra is our true foundation of compassion as it is love expressed that becomes compassion.

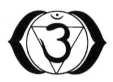

sixth chakra: third eye chakra

Sanskrit name: Ajna

Position: Between the eyebrows

Color: Purple/violet

Crystal: Amethyst

Endocrine gland: Pituitary

Physical region: Eyes, ears, nose, and skeletal system

Life aspect: Truthful perception, spiritual vision, wisdom, imagination, deepest intuition, and a sense of the unknown.

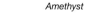

Amethyst

Third eye chakra in balance: Helps remove confusion and perceive the self and world with clarity, good judgment, and wisdom. Promotes a calm reassurance and definition of life's path and authenticity.

seventh chakra: crown chakra

Sanskrit name: Sahasrara or Adhipati

Position: Top of the head

Color: White

Crystal: Quartz

Endocrine gland: Pineal

Physical region: Head, brain, and nervous system

Life Aspect: This chakra links the individual and the universal, aids the connection with the higher self and the divine, elevates spirituality, and gives us evolved judgment.

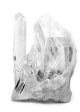

Quartz

Crown chakra in balance: Helps relieve loneliness and reminds us of our connection with all that is one. Allows for expanded awareness on an emotional level, and a sense of connected wisdom.

chakras—making the connection

To me chakras are never blocked but only in need of motivating or "jump-starting." They are receptors of universal energy, feeding us inspiration, power, and creativity, without which we can become depleted and ineffectual in the world. This energy is as vital to the auric body as food is to the physical body.

1 Begin with the first or root/base chakra at the base of the spine. See a beautiful red swirling vortex with an open rose at its tip. Think of this chakra connecting the body to the earth. This chakra is linked with issues of identity and boundary.

2 Next, focus on the second or sacral chakra between the navel and genitals. See a beautiful swirling orange vortex with an orange flower petal open at its tip. This center relates to intuition, inner wisdom, knowing, trust, and loving the inner self.

3 Now the third or solar plexus chakra just below the breastbone or sternum. See a swirling yellow vortex with a silky yellow flower at its tip. This center relates to one's personal power and continued sense of innocence and adventure. See a vibrant yellow color enter this chakra.

4 The heart chakra is located between the nipples. See a glowing, swirling, bright green vortex with a beautiful green flower at its tip. The heart chakra is the center of love and compassion. Watch as the green becomes more vibrant.

5 Focus on the throat chakra. See a deep blue vortex in the area of the throat. This chakra is the center of communication, compassion, and love. It also helps to clarify your direction in life. See the vibrant blue growing stronger and brighter.

6 The third eye or brow chakra is located in the middle of your forehead. See a purple swirling flower. The brow chakra is the center of insight and wisdom. Fill this vortex with the most beautiful velvety purple and enjoy the bliss it brings.

7 The seventh or crown chakra encircles the top or your head and expands to a palm's width above your head. See a swirling white vortex with a lily at its end. This chakra is our place of bliss and connection with the sacred prana of the universe and creator—in whatever form that takes for us. Enjoy this sense of expansion.

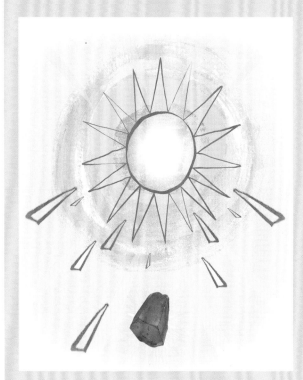

auric shower

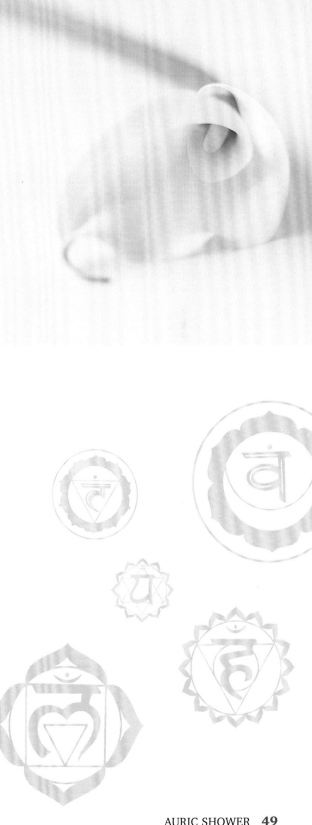

I call this meditation an auric shower, as it washes the energetic system. Just as doctors wash their hands before treating a patient, I have an "energetic shower" before or after a day's healing. This meditation can also help if I am feeling negative for some reason.

I often meditate just before I have a cup of peppermint tea, sitting by the beach. We are all like sponges, picking up other people's negative thoughts throughout the day, through radio waves, mobile phone conversations, and other people's attitudes. Just as we wash our body everyday with soap and water, cleansing away the accumulated grime of the day, so can we wash our "auric" systems with pure energy to rid ourselves of any negative energy. Yet so many people neglect this liberating form of cleansing.

This auric shower meditation helps clear the negative residue that can result from modern life. You can spend up to 50 minutes on this a day, but just five minutes can make all the difference. Think of it as having a shower of light, after a stressful day spent with a draining or negative friend, or in a busy city street or a crowded train, filled with others' negative thoughts, or any event that left you angry, sad, or residing in the negative part of your psyche. Thomas Moore, the author of *Care of the Soul*, talked about how we care for our physical bodies but not our souls. This meditation will help you care for your soul, or inner self, and that of others.

auric shower visualization

A Vietnamese Buddhist monk I trained with years ago always began the class with ten minutes of "smiling meditation." I would like you to begin this visualization by smiling.

1 To start, sit comfortably in an upright chair. Sit well into the chair so that your lower back is supported, backs of your thighs firmly on the seat, knees apart, and hands resting on your upper thighs, palms down. Have your eyes closed and your face in a relaxed smile.

2 Now breathe in and out through your nose normally. At the same time, silently count each in-breath till you reach ten and then start again at one. This will begin to center and focus you. If you lose count, don't worry, just start again.

3 Now imagine your own personal ideal of nature—such as a beautiful beach at sunset with the waves lapping at your feet or a tranquil forest with the sun streaming through the leaves as you sit on a smooth warm log. Make this your "internal screen saver" and come back to it every day. You will find that you build up the energy of this internal space, making it easier and easier to access each day.

4 After you have focused on your breath for as long as feels comfortable, begin to visualize with each in-breath that you are breathing in peace, love, tranquility, health, and clarity of thought. With each out-breath, visualize that you are exhaling any accumulated stress, anxiety, or negativity. Imagine you have a beautiful damask rose before you and are gently breathing in its exquisite scent, silently repeating the following with each in-breath, "I am inhaling peace, love, and tranquility" and silently repeating with each out-breath, "I am exhaling any physical stress or emotional tension." Repeat this for as long as feels comfortable (say, around 20 times). Imagine you are inhaling and exhaling with your whole body.

5 Now imagine a Perspex tube emerging from the base of your spine and going right down into mother earth. Begin to see any residual negativity being flushed out of you and into this Perspex tube. See yourself letting go of any accumulated stress, negative thought patterns, or any physical injuries or illnesses. This is a good way to rid yourself of aches and pains, too. I like to imagine four or five vacuum pipes appearing to suck away any dusty film that has become stuck to me. I see these pipes going down into mother earth carrying the energetic debris, to be transformed and revitalized into positive energy.

6 Once I feel my system is clearer, I begin to see the top of my head open, and a funnel of light pour into me. See it fill your head, eyes, ears, cheeks, neck, and throat, upper back, heart, and lungs, then your shoulders, upper arms, elbows, hands, fingers, and chest. Feel your diaphragm relax with this beautiful golden light. Feel your solar plexus, stomach, intestines, hips, and spine all breathe in this healing warm sunshine, then your sacrum, your reproductive system, thighs, knees, calves, ankles, feet, and toes.

7 Feel your whole body glow. Imagine you become the sunshine and are glowing. Each cell is filled with peace, love, and tranquility. As you sit there glowing, I would like you to make contact with your chakras (see page 48).

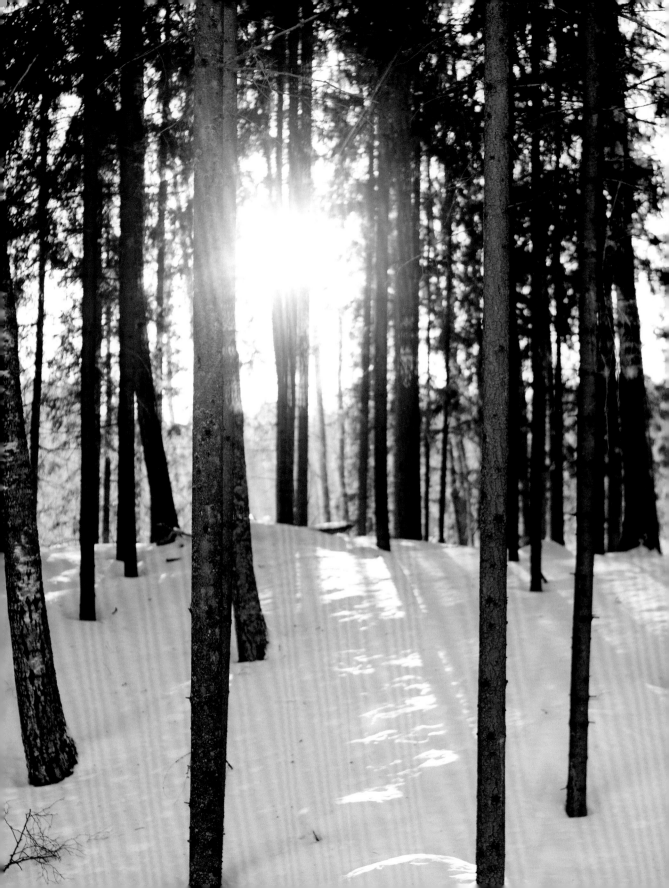

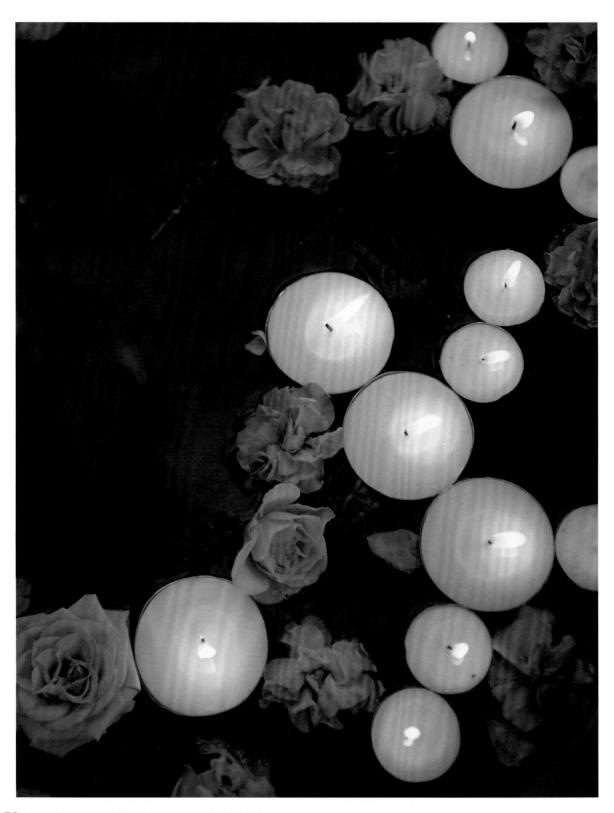

8 See all the chakras go right through your body, front and back. Imagine these chakras have dials and increase the level of intensity so that they all resonate at the same height. Imagine the chakras acting as receptors for universal energy and light, filling you with creative vigor, vitality, clarity, and wisdom.

9 If you have any issues that are reflected in one or more of the chakras that need focus in your life, you could think of concentrating on those chakras. Imagine more of the color associated with each of those chakras pouring into it as you would pour water on a thirsty plant. Imagine those chakras reviving and glowing. Don't worry if this seems an effort at first. Focus on the power of your thought and patiently repeat this with patient intention and all is possible.

10 Finally, I like to give thanks for this sense of renewed peace. You can choose who you would like to give that thanks to, depending on your own personal beliefs. I give thanks to the universe and goddess. I am sure it will get to the right place somehow.

11 End by coming to, slowly, taking time to reconnect with your physical body. If you feel like it, and you have time, rest afterwards. I often feel invigorated and ready to begin or continue the day. Better than any cup of coffee!

I have described the full meditation. Feel free to use any parts of it you choose. For example, if you only have five minutes to spare, you could start with the "smiling meditation" and then progress to the "Perspex tube." If you have more time available, you can do more of it. Record this meditation and listen to it when you have a quiet moment.

You will find that, with practice, the auric shower will become quicker and quicker to do, so it is worth doing the whole meditation several times so that your system knows the route well and you will get to this relaxed, clear space in no time at all. After all, time is relative and change can happen in a passing second!

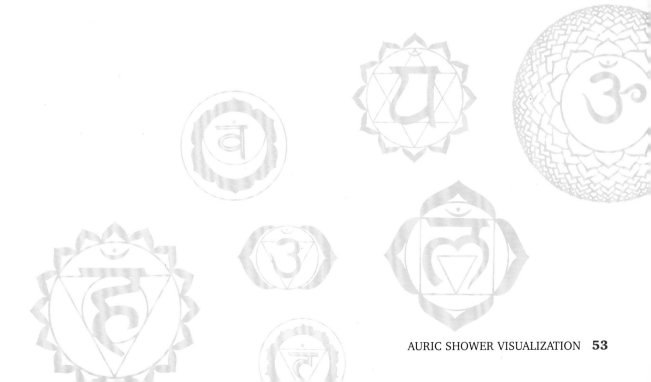

healing hands visualization

The calm period after the auric shower is the perfect time to create your energetic healing hands.

I suggest that after you come to, slowly, imagine you are holding in your hands a tennis ball-size sphere of golden light. See it, feel it, cup it in your hands, and look at it. Start by expanding this tennis ball gently. As you pull your hands apart, begin to feel the warmth as if actually holding a ball of golden light. See light coming out of your hands and creating this ball. Pull your hands wider apart while still maintaining a sense of contact with the ball of energy between your hands. Feel the energy come out of your hands. This is good preparation for giving healing to yourself or others.

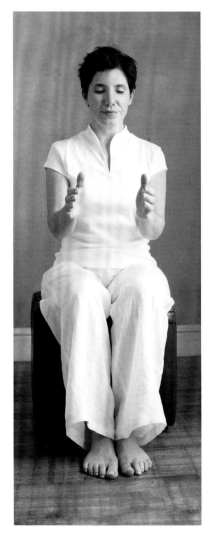
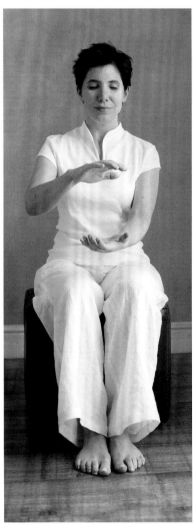

Before giving a healing treatment, energize your hands. Visualize a glowing ball of light and let your hands trace its form.

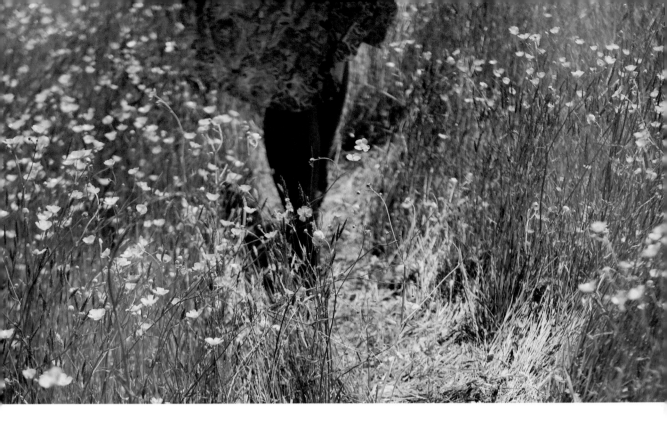

the gift of healing

To me, healing means channeling your compassion, love, and care into others. It is no different from a kind word said to a stranger. An ability to make someone feel better is not an exclusively mystical experience, needing years of training and deep faith. It is about the natural ability we all have—should we wish to nurture it. There is healing everywhere. I always say my car mechanic is a very genuine kind of healer! To help you focus your healing powers, imagine the rays of sunshine on a beautiful summer's day pouring out of your hands to help someone. If you "intend" to help someone you have significantly more power than you can ever imagine, the power of imagined love or light entering your body to heal. Something as simple and free as that can begin to change your life and open up a new pathway for you.

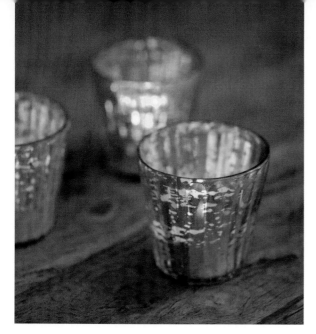

Create an ambiance for healing with calming music and gentle lighting. Candles give off a calm, natural light, evoking a serenity perfect for healing.

preparation for giving healing

Make sure you really feel like giving some healing at this time. If you are tired or stressed it would be best to postpone it for another time. Never give healing out of a feeling of obligation or responsibility. It is a gift to be given, as was once described to me in a workshop from the center of compassion communication, only if you can do so with "the joy of a child feeding a hungry duck" or, as I often say, "as a happy dog running towards the ocean with his stick."

Prepare the space by making the room lovely. Include some flowers, a candle, a warm blanket to cover the recipient, a comfortable clean pillow, and an aromatherapy burner with frankincense and lavender. An extra touch would be to play some tranquil meditation music. A massage table is ideal but if you do not have one, then a bed with a chair at a comfortable height for you to sit on is just as good. An alternative, depending on how flexible you are, would be to place a thick quilt on the floor and make yourself comfortable sitting on a cushion

placed on the floor at one end. Remember that intention is everything. Trust your intention. Wash your hands with soap and water before you start and as you do so, imagine all the negative residues of the day are being washed away, as if in a fresh mountain stream. Imagine the water washing over your whole body.

Seated comfortably, perform the auric shower meditation. You could do this together, if the recipient is willing. Or you could read the meditation to the recipient in a slow, calm voice, guiding them through the auric shower or chakra meditation. This, in itself, is a very powerful tool of intention and healing. Then ask the recipient to lie down on their back comfortably on the bed, table, or a quilt you have prepared.

Ask the recipient if there is anything they would like you to concentrate on. Their answers may give you some idea of what parts of the body you might like to focus on, or which chakras might need extra attention. Ask them to let you know if they feel hot or cold or uncomfortable during the healing. If you are playing some music, check that they like the music you selected. Ensure that the volume is okay for them, too.

giving a healing

Before you begin, gently place your hands on the recipient's head. I often place my first fingers gently at the opening of their ears. This is inspired by a cranial sacral technique I learned many years ago. You are now ready to begin the healing.

1 Imagine you are holding the ball of light. Visualize it passing through the top of your head, through your chest and arms and into your hands. Now see it pour into the recipient's head, then through their body.

2 Visualize this universal light of love and peace filling you both. Become aware of any areas that "feel" different in any way, while you imagine light filling the recipient. Allow this to form in your mind's eye. Often mysteriously, this will give a very accurate indication of problem areas. Focus the light on any areas that the recipient has previously mentioned, or to which you feel naturally drawn. Simply doing this can sometimes be enough to elicit positive results. Continue visualizing light until you are satisfied that these compressed areas are released or will continue to free themselves as you move on. Do this for as long as you need to send light throughout their whole body.

3 Now focus on your hands, and imagine you are drawing the light back into them. Now very, very slowly, take your hands away. During this kind of healing, the whole auric system slows down immensely. You need to support this new, slower rhythm, so move slowly and quietly as if wading through a beautiful mountain lake or trying not to wake a baby. Loud sounds can startle the recipient at this stage.

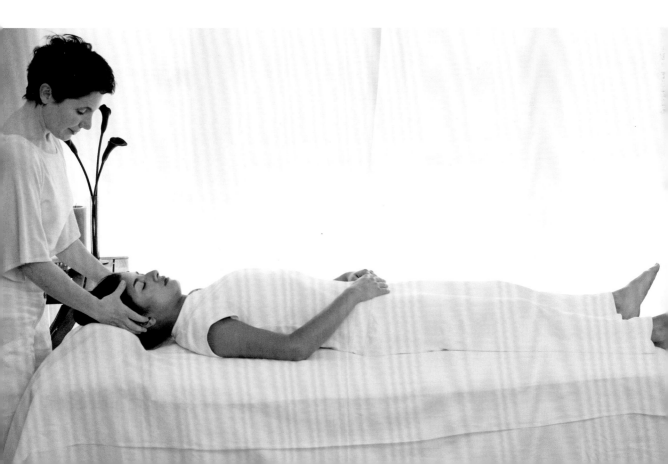

4 Slowly walk round to the side of the recipient. Place your hand about one palm-width above each chakra, visualizing the colors and strength of each one. If a chakra "feels" different (in temperature, or you just have an inexplicable feeling) spend some time visualizing a vibrant chakra, using the image of golden light motivating the vortex. See the color that relates to each chakra (see pages 44–48).

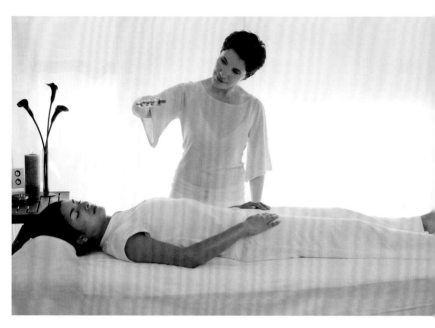

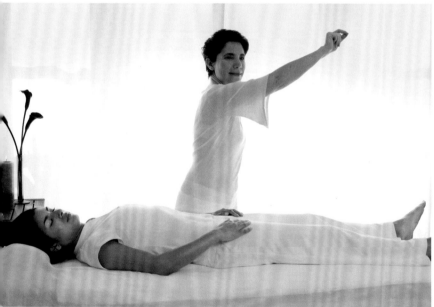

5 When you have gone over each of the seven chakras with your palm, snap your fingers three times in the air around the head and into the aura. This clears the energy. Then snap your fingers around the lower part of the body. This helps to release energy that may have gathered at the recipient's feet.

6 Allow your hands to gently waft onto the recipient's feet and lightly hold. Stay there for a few moments to help the person reconnect with the earth and become grounded again. This helps prevent them becoming too "spaced out."

7 Sometimes I use a set of chimes to ring out once or twice to clear the energy. You can use Tibetan bells (right), or a rain stick. As hearing is the first sense to develop in the womb and the last to go when we die, hearing beautiful frequencies can be a very powerful clearing ending to a healing session.

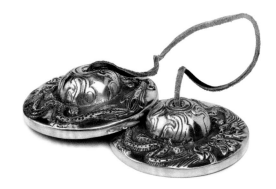

8 Tell the recipient you hope they enjoyed your healing and silently wish them peace, love, and clarity. Tell them to relax and come to slowly and say you will be back in a few moments. Now quietly leave the room to wash your hands under lots of running water. Imagine the water washes away any energetic residue that does not belong to you. Imagine the water washing you from head to toe. Drink a glass of water and give one to the recipient when you return.

Once the healing is over and the room returns to its normal function, open the window and light a stick of incense to clear any potential energetic residue, and signify the true end of the session. Your wellbeing is of paramount importance too. Usually, I feel energized and vital after a healing session and hopefully so will you. If you feel drained, rest a while and have a warming herbal tea. Remember that you should not attempt to give a healing when you are tired, anxious, hungry, or ill at ease. Always prepare yourself first or save this wonderful, shared experience for another day. Blessings.

USING CRYSTALS

This is the perfect time to use a crystal for a chakra that needs balancing. See pages 44–48 on chakras, healing crystals, and their meanings. Be creative, be instinctive and you will know. Hold the crystal above the chakra and about 1ft (30cm) away. Allow the power of the crystal, its own energy and properties, as well as your intention to activate and empower. Ask silently that the recipient's own wisdom takes what it needs here.

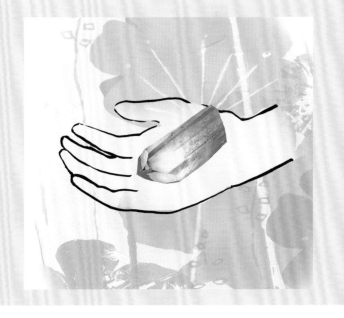

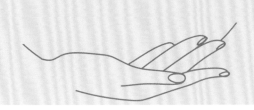

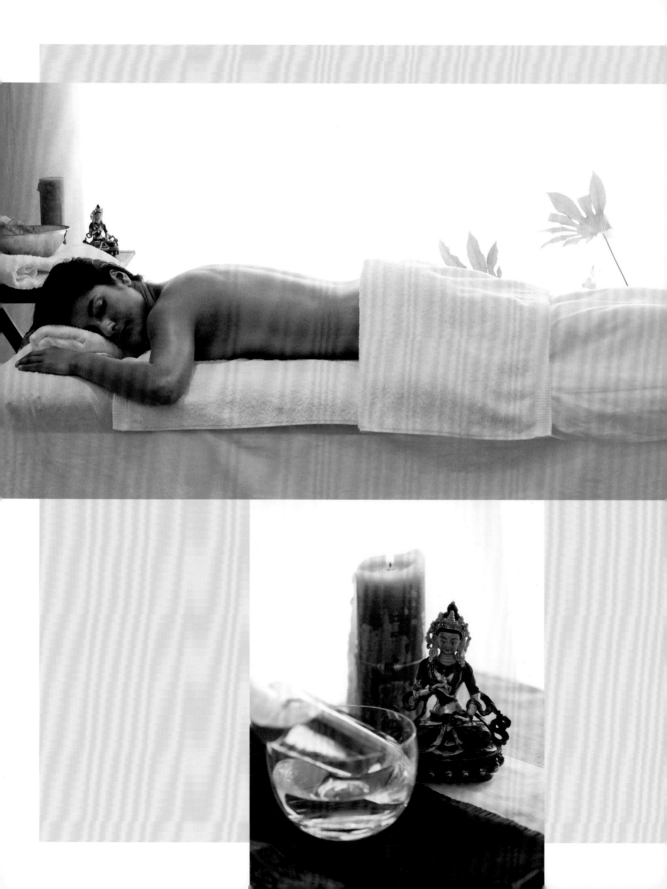

ayurveda

India and Ayurveda have long been a significant part of my cultural mix. My father was born in India and introduced me to many of the Ayurvedic rituals of lifestyle and diet. My first experience of giving a healing massage was when I was about six years old, relieving my father's back pain by trampling my feet as hard as I could along his back and legs as he lay on the floor. Years later I began my own journey into the wisdom and knowledge of Ayurvedic massage. I felt an instant affinity with Ayurvedic medicine and have integrated many of its concepts into my personal lifestyle, practices, and philosophy of life.

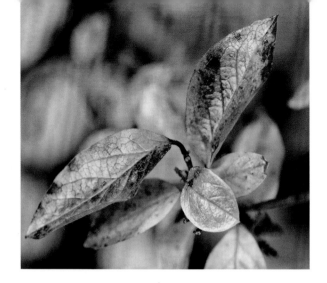

what is ayurveda?

Ayurveda originated in India over 3,000 years ago. Ayurvedic principles greatly influenced both the Ancient Greek and Traditional Chinese forms of medicine. In India's ancient Sanskrit language, Ayurveda means the "science or knowledge of life." It is a holistic philosophy that integrates body, mind, spirit, and universal energy, and is based on the principle that by achieving balance you can maintain harmony and peace of mind and so prevent disease.

According to Ayurvedic philosophy, everything in life—people, animals, disease, food, and the universe itself—are made up of three main energetic elements, or "Doshas," namely Vata (air), Pitta (fire), and Kapha (earth). It is the unique balance, or Doshic mix, of two or more of these elements that gives us our individuality. The Doshas are responsible for a person's "Prakruti," or constitution, including mental and emotional nature, as well as their physical characteristics, such as build, color of hair, skin tone and texture, color, shape and size of eyes, sleep patterns, preferred tastes, and any medical symptoms.

A simple way to understand the difference between the three Doshas, I find, is through Ayurvedic pulse diagnosis. A Vata pulse is like the snake—long, thin, quick, and cold. The

Pitta pulse is like the frog—exuberant, determined, active, joyful, bounding, and loud. The Kapha pulse is like the swan—slow, graceful, thoughtful, and sometimes inactively awaiting its swan song. Most people have a Doshic mix of one or two Doshas and some are "tri-Doshic" and have all three in balance.

The beauty of Ayurveda is its belief that the Doshas can and do change their dominance. They can go in and out of balance, depending on how we live our lives, our age and life experiences, and even the seasons. The responsibility is given to us to achieve balance through herbs and treatment and by adopting a "Sattvik" lifestyle—one that is lived calmly and in harmony with ourselves and our deepest physical, spiritual, emotional, and creative needs.

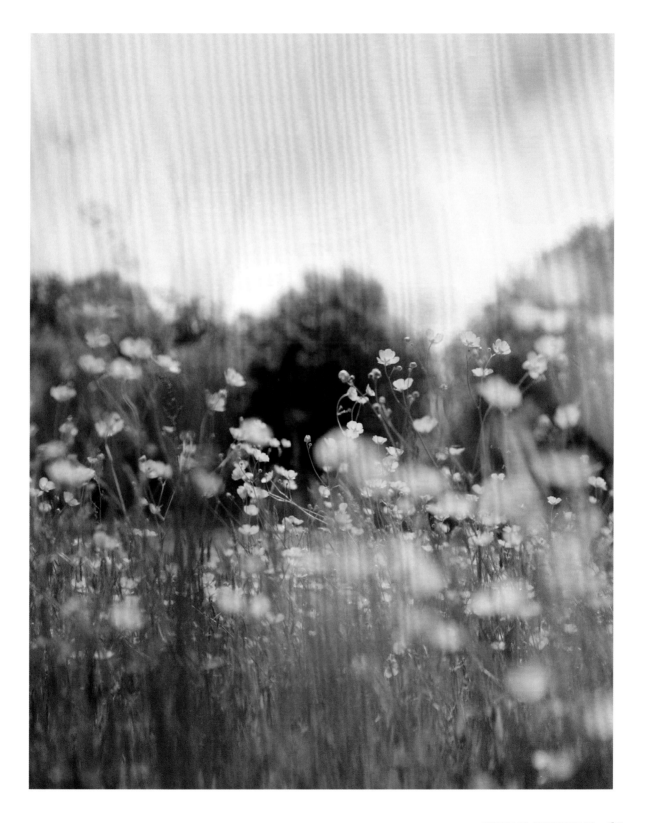

which dosha are you?

To access the wisdom, ideology, and techniques of Ayurvedic healing, complete this questionnaire to find which of your Doshas is most prominent:

Kapha, Pitta, or Vata. Tick the questions that best describe you, then see the Doshic profiles on pages 66–67.

Vata

☐ Thin, and usually always have been, can be tall or short, light bones

☐ Small, active, dark eyes

☐ Dry skin, chaps easily

☐ Prefer warm climate, moisture

☐ Dark, rough, kinky hair

☐ Variable appetite

☐ Bowel movements irregular, hard, dry

☐ Digestion sometimes good

☐ Dislike routine

☐ Creative thinker

☐ Like to stay physically active

☐ Mentally relaxed when exercising

☐ Change your mind easily

☐ Tend towards fear or anxiety under stress

☐ Often dream, but rarely remember your dreams

☐ Changeable moods and ideas

☐ Like to snack, nibble

☐ If ill, nervous disorders or sharp pain

☐ Light sleeper

☐ You think that money is there to be spent

☐ Brittle nails

☐ Cold hands and feet, little perspiration

☐ Thin, fast, variable pulse, hands cold

☐ Variable thirst

Pitta

☐ Medium, well-proportioned frame, can gain or lose weight easily

☐ Penetrating light green, grey, or amber eyes

☐ Fair skin, sunburn easily

☐ Prefer cool, well-ventilated places

☐ Fine, light oily hair, blond, red, or early grey

☐ Good appetite

☐ Easy and regular bowel activity

☐ Usually good digestion

☐ Enjoy planning and like routine

☐ Good initiator and leader

☐ Enjoy physical activities

☐ Exercise helps keep emotions from going out of control

☐ Have opinions to share

☐ Tend towards anger, frustration, or irritability under stress

☐ Relatively easy to remember your dreams, often in color

☐ Forceful about expressing ideas and feelings

☐ Like high-protein foods

☐ If ill, fevers, rash, inflammation

☐ Usually sleep well

☐ You think that money is best spent on special items or on purchases that advance you

☐ Flexible nails, but pretty strong

☐ Good circulation, perspire a lot

☐ Strong full pulse, hands warm

☐ Usually thirsty

Kapha

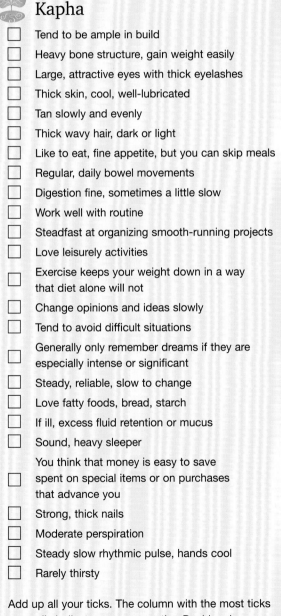

- [ ] Tend to be ample in build
- [ ] Heavy bone structure, gain weight easily
- [ ] Large, attractive eyes with thick eyelashes
- [ ] Thick skin, cool, well-lubricated
- [ ] Tan slowly and evenly
- [ ] Thick wavy hair, dark or light
- [ ] Like to eat, fine appetite, but you can skip meals
- [ ] Regular, daily bowel movements
- [ ] Digestion fine, sometimes a little slow
- [ ] Work well with routine
- [ ] Steadfast at organizing smooth-running projects
- [ ] Love leisurely activities
- [ ] Exercise keeps your weight down in a way that diet alone will not
- [ ] Change opinions and ideas slowly
- [ ] Tend to avoid difficult situations
- [ ] Generally only remember dreams if they are especially intense or significant
- [ ] Steady, reliable, slow to change
- [ ] Love fatty foods, bread, starch
- [ ] If ill, excess fluid retention or mucus
- [ ] Sound, heavy sleeper
- [ ] You think that money is easy to save spent on special items or on purchases that advance you
- [ ] Strong, thick nails
- [ ] Moderate perspiration
- [ ] Steady slow rhythmic pulse, hands cool
- [ ] Rarely thirsty

Add up all your ticks. The column with the most ticks generally indicates your presenting Doshic mix.

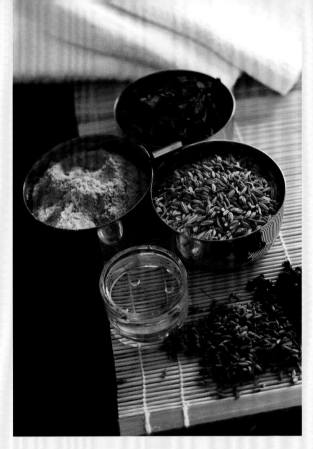

In Ayurveda, scrubs and oil blends are adjusted according to your dominant Dosha.

ACHIEVING HARMONY

Ayurvedic practitioners believe that the root of all disease is "Asantosa," or dissatisfaction and disharmony with the universal forces. A good, healthy, long life can be attained through personal harmony with our deepest physical, emotional, creative, and spiritual needs, achieved through a supportive diet, exercise routine, regular sleep, meditation practice, and harmony with the elemental clock of day, season, and age.

your doshic constitution

vata

The physical manifestation of the Vata type is of tall, slender, or skinny build, fine hair, and "bead-like" pupils. In balance, the Vata-dominant person has a strong nervous system, efficient metabolism, and healthy digestive system.

However, factors such as emotional strain, diet, environment, travel, old age, excessive exercise, or prolonged sense of insecurity may lead to imbalance in the Vata personality. Out of balance, the Vata person might have dry skin, cold hands and feet, and digestive problems.

On the mental level, the balanced Vata personality would be expressed through creativity, intuition, artistry, and spiritual depth. Out of balance, this same energy would be seen as doubt, insecurity, paranoia, and over-sensitivity to the environment. The emotional manifestations of the balanced Vata individual would be exhilaration, intuition, and a higher sense of peace. Out of balance, the Vata type would show fear, insecurity, and anxiety.

vata pacifying steps

Eat foods that contain warming spices such as ginger, chili, and cumin. Drink warm fluids. Take vigorous exercise such as aerobics or cycling. Keep warm and get adequate rest. Have Abhyanga (see page 68).

pitta

The physical manifestation of the Pitta type is of a medium build that is generally well-proportioned and muscular, blue or hazel almond-shaped eyes and blond/red or prematurely grey hair. In balance, a Pitta-dominant person would have a strong digestion, heart, and liver. However, factors such as spicy foods, summer heat, excessive exercise, and stressful or angry situations may lead to imbalance in a Pitta type.

Out of balance, a Pitta person may have symptoms of excess heat, such as skin inflammation, ulcers, acne, rash, or eczema, and hot flushes. The balanced Pitta personality would be expressed with intelligence, confidence, charisma, and sharp wit. Out of balance, this same energy would be expressed as domineering behavior, sarcasm, and a tendency to be overly critical. In balance, the emotional manifestation of the Pitta type would be excitement, joy, courage, and a penetrating heart. Out of balance, this would become irritability, anger, impatience, and jealousy.

pitta pacifying steps

Eat meals little and often. Do not allow yourself to get too hungry. Avoid stimulants such as alcohol and coffee. Avoid spicy foods. Take moderate exercise in cool air, such as moonlight walks and gardening. Have Abhyanga (see page 68) with a Pitta pacifying blend.

kapha

The physical manifestation of the Kapha type is of a rounded or overweight build, big smile, teeth and lips, dark brown hair, and pale, oily, or lustrous complexion, relatively heavy hips and legs, and a quiet calmness.

In balance a Kapha person has a good memory, strong chest and lungs, and muscular build, with slow, graceful movements. Out of balance, a Kapha person would be overweight, cold, with fluid retention and digestive bloating. On a mental level, the balanced Kapha would be a good decision maker, devoted to friends and family, and with a tranquil nature. Out of balance, this same energy would be exhibited as mental inertia and over-attachment.

The emotional manifestation of the Kapha type in balance would be an affectionate, patient, and sympathetic personality. Out of balance, this would become greed, lethargy, depression, self-sabotage, and a tendency towards addictive behavior. Factors such as cold sugary foods, winter cold, lack of physical activity or exercise, and allowing greed or attachment to reign free may affect the Kapha type.

kapha pacifying steps

Reduce intake of sugar and cold foods. Drink warming fluids. Keep warm. Stimulate the body with a full body Utvartana dry massage (see page 87). Engage in regular, vigorous exercise and rise to any challenge that motivates you. Have Abhyanga (see page 68).

Vata types can eat warming, spicy foods (top) while Pitta types should avoid spices (center). Kapha types should keep plenty of warming fluids on hand (right).

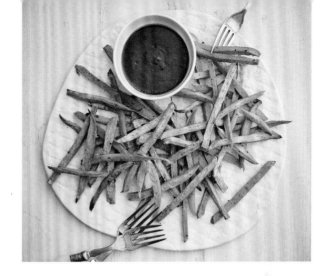

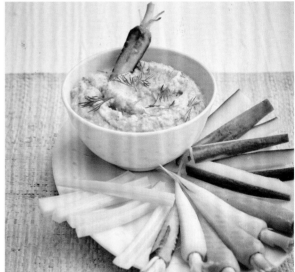

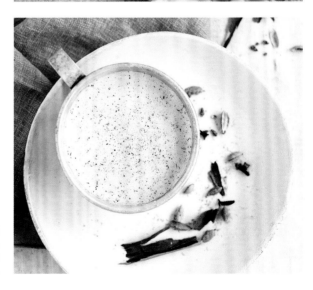

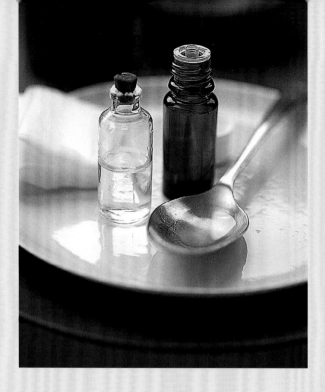

abhyanga—the ayurvedic massage

Ayurvedic massage—Abhyanga—is a highly individual treatment designed to ease mind and body and promote a deep sense of peace and relaxation. I use a luxurious heated oil plus massage techniques specially tailored to the individual's needs and designed to act as a catalyst to the person's own healing processes. The massage strokes are chosen to suit the recipient's Doshic mix. For example, long and slow movements for a Vata-dominant person, quick and stimulating strokes for a Kapha-dominant type, or a mixture of massage styles for the Pitta-dominant individual. Additionally, I use special Ayurvedic essential oil blends to help balance the recipient's presenting Dosha.

aromatherapy and ayurveda—the blends

I use two to three 9fl oz (250ml) bottles of massage oil for each Abhyanga, on average. A significant part of the pleasure of this massage is the copious amounts of oil you use. You'll be amazed at how much oil the skin absorbs, giving a wonderfully relaxing and luxurious feeling. You can use any suitable massage oil, such as sweet almond or sunflower oil. Add eight drops in total of the following essential oils to each 9fl oz (250ml) bottle of massage oil, according to the predominant Dosha:

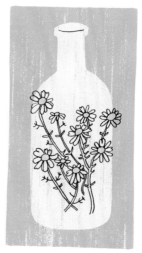

Pitta: Rose, sandalwood, or chamomile
Vata: Cedarwood, eucalyptus, or ylang ylang
Kapha: Ginger, lemongrass, or rosemary

Place the bottle of oil in a metal container filled with hot water to warm it. Always test the oil to make sure it is warm enough—but not too hot—before applying. For a full massage, three bottles of oil are recommended for Pitta- and Vata-dominant individuals. For the Kapha type, use no more than two bottles of oil, as too much can aggravate the Kapha Dosha and would be counterproductive (see the Utvartana box on page 87).

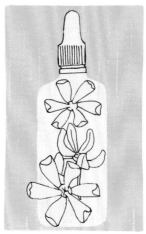

An herbal bath makes a lovely complement to any home Abhyanga (see page 70), or you could add a few drops of each essential oil to the bath. Always agitate the water to mix the oils well and take care to avoid dropping essential oil directly onto your skin, as ginger or rosemary in particular can cause skin irritation.

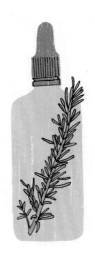

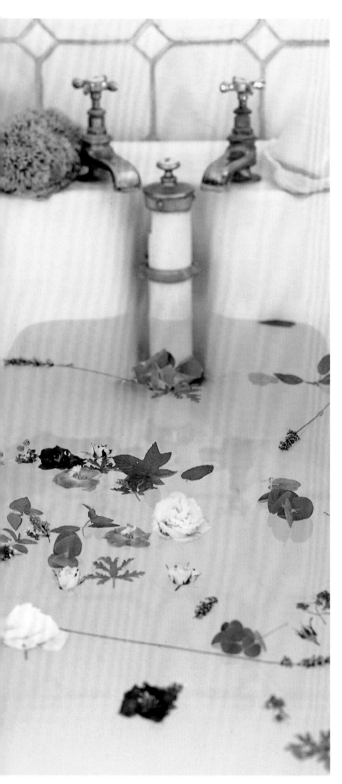

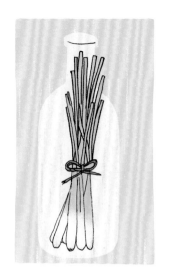

ayurvedic herbal bath

An Ayurvedic herbal bath is a lovely way to relax, re-energize, and rebalance before or after an Abhyanga. To make one, take a piece of muslin cloth and fill it with herbs according to the Dosha in need of balancing (see below) then fold it up and twist it into a tight knot. Tie the top with string and soak in a hot running bath (not too hot for Pitta-dominant types).

Vata: Fresh rosemary and eucalyptus leaves
Pitta: Dried rose and lavender
Kapha: Fresh ginger and lemongrass

Vata and Kapha types should have 15-minute herbal bath treatments, and 10 minutes for Pitta types.

ayurvedic massage techniques

During the Abhyanga, or massage, adapt your massage strokes to the dominant Dosha type of the recipient, as follows:

Vata: Apply light, slow, deliberate, smoothing, gentle, soothing rhythmic strokes. The copious amount of oil used in an Ayurvedic massage acts as a barrier for the sensitive Vata skin and provides a sense of protection from the external world.

Pitta: Apply medium pressure and a mixture of slow, deliberate smoothing strokes, of varying speeds and rhythms. This variation is designed to occupy the highly active Pitta mind and thus aid relaxation.

Kapha: Apply deeper pressure and a more dynamic, invigorating massage that is much quicker and stronger than for Vata- or Pitta-dominant individuals, the rubbing movements giving extra friction to aid circulation and dispel sluggishness. Use less oil for Kapha types, and perhaps dry brushing for some of the time (see page 87).

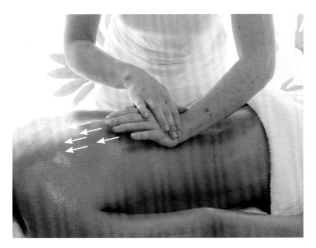

1 heel-of-hand pushes

Using the heel of one palm, push up the back assisted by the other hand to provide extra pressure. Apply deep pressure for the Kapha type, a mixture of deep and light for a Pitta-dominant person, and lightly and slowly for the Vata individual.

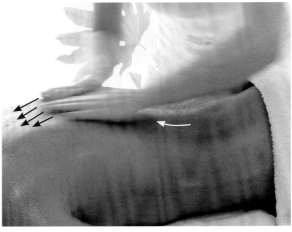

2 double-palm oiling

This technique enhances absorption of the oil and so allows deep lubrication of the body. The move can be performed very slowly for the Vata type, a mixture of slow and fast for a Pitta individual and more quickly and invigoratingly for a Kapha-dominant person.

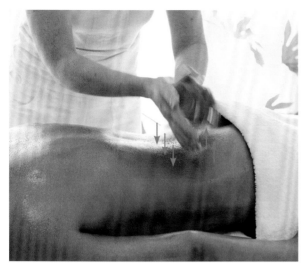

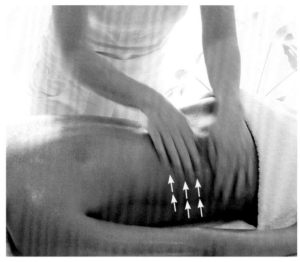

3 light chopping

In this stroke the hands work alternately, making light chopping movements to stimulate the area. This stroke is suitable for the Pitta and Kapha types.

4 pull ups

In this stroke, the hands alternately pull up the sides towards the back. Do this slowly for a Vata type, use a mixture of slow and fast movements for a Pitta individual, and quickly for the Kapha-dominant.

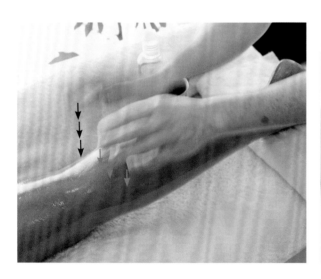

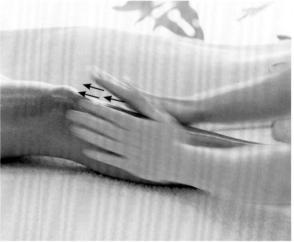

5 tapping

Here the hands tap the body rhythmically, as though lightly playing a drum. It is suitable for Pitta and Kapha types.

6 double-handed rubs

For this stroke, rub the hands simultaneously along the leg in sets of five, as follows: ankle to knee, knee to top of thigh, and front and back of legs. Vary the speed according to Dosha: Kapha—quick and stimulating, Vata—slow and deliberate, and Pitta—a mix of the two.

abhyanga: head

First, prepare the treatment table. You will need a sheet, three towels (one to support the head), a pillow, and massage oil. Warm the bottles of oil in advance—two or three 9fl oz (250ml) bottles according to Dosha-dominant type. Have a container of hot water nearby to keep the bottles warm.

An Abhyanga massage pays special attention to head, face, abdomen, feet, and especially joints. Ask the recipient to lie on their back, face upwards. Place a pillow under their knees and a small, folded towel under the nape of their neck. Before you start, make the sound "aum" (the first sound of creation) together, or ring Tibetan bells three times, slowly and deliberately.

This first sequence is the Abhyanga of the head (oiling of the head). When you have finished this

sequence, cover the recipient's head with a towel to keep warm and allow the oil to penetrate the hair and scalp. I really like this step as it feels so cozy and cocoon-like.

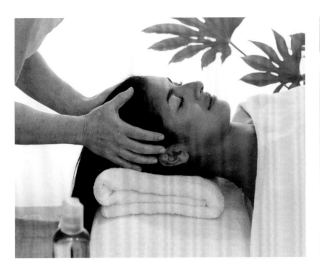

1 Using both hands, hold the head of the recipient with palms on top of the head, always thinking of transmitting love, peace, and Pranic energy.

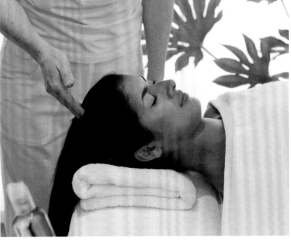

2 Start with the crown chakra, Adhipati. Prana or divine energy is believed to accumulate in the head so beginning here releases the energy throughout the body and prepares the Pranic channel to be more receptive.

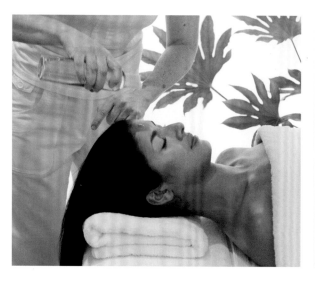

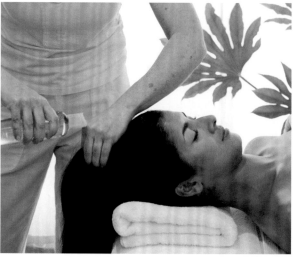

3 Carefully pour the warmed oil onto the third eye chakra, Ajna, maintaining a gentle stream. The flow of warm oil over this important chakra is very calming to the spirit. Maintain your focus here, keeping a steady stream of oil.

4 Again, pouring carefully, saturate the hair completely and massage the head all over. This warm oil not only feels wonderful and nourishes the hair, it also calms the spirit. I put a towel on the floor underneath the head to catch any drips of oil.

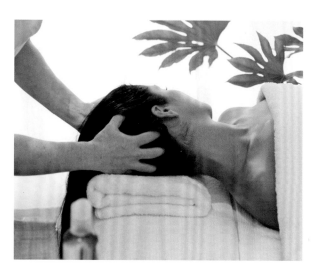

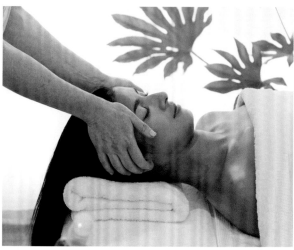

5 Turn the recipient's head to the side so that you can massage the side of their head. Administer more warm oil here, as it feels so relaxing.

6 Using the soft part of each of your palms, very gently massage the recipient's forehead from the center outwards and downwards. This improves memory and alertness and balances the pituitary and pineal glands.

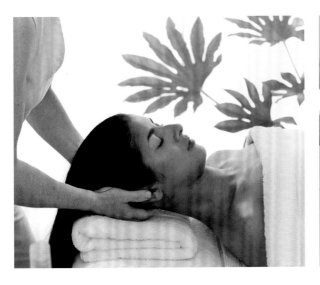

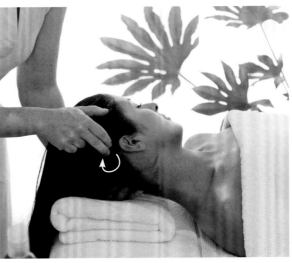

7 Lift the head slightly and press the area where the head and neck meet. Now press, just using your fingertips, alternating your right and left hands. This step balances the nervous system and helps promote stability.

8 Using your first and second finger, massage the area just behind the tip of the ear in very small clockwise movements. This stimulates the Marma point, or energy vortex (see introduction, page 78) which helps to balance the intestines and thought processes.

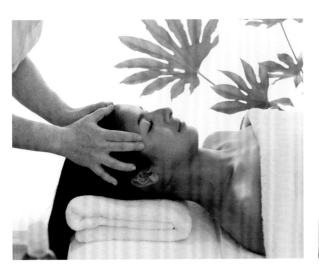

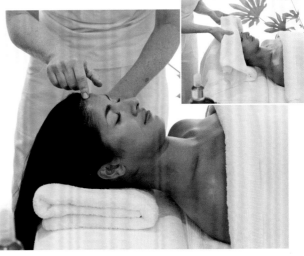

9 Using your first and second fingers again, lightly rub the temples. This balances the mind and inspires creativity.

10 Using your first finger only, press an invisible line from the third eye chakra, Ajna, in the center of the forehead, along the midline of the head to the crown chakra, Adhipati. This move deepens our connection with divine Pranic energy and aids spiritual insights.

abhyanga: front upper body and arms

In this sequence we work on the upper body, arms, and hands, which are especially rich in energy points. You can top up the metal container with hot water at this point to make sure that the massage oil is being kept at the right temperature.

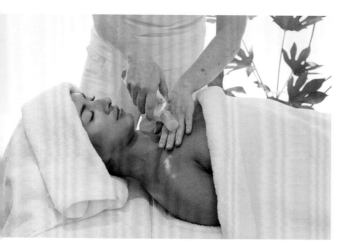

1 Start this sequence by oiling the top of the chest and shoulders, using the Ayurvedic technique of carefully pouring the oil over your hand. The warm oil soothes and relaxes as you pour.

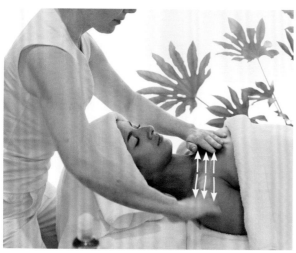

2 Using your right hand and then left, as shown, massage across the top of the chest to really lubricate this area with oil, employing appropriate strokes according to the recipient's Doshic type.

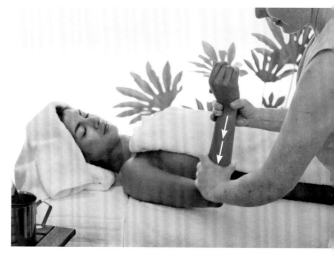

3 Holding the recipient's arm at the wrist with your right hand, massage with your left hand using a downward pushing and squeezing movement, as if gently wringing water out of a cloth. The warm oil allows your hand to glide easily along the arm.

4 Hold the recipient's arm at the wrist with your left hand and interlace your fingers with their fingers. Now gently flex and extend their wrist. This relieves any tension in the lower arm and wrist.

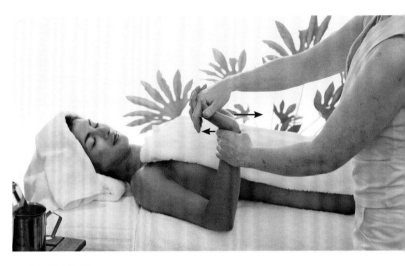

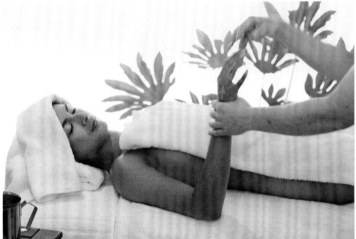

5 Continue to hold their wrist with your left hand and gently sweep and pull upwards over their fingers. The hands are rich in energy points and this activates them, balancing all the Marma points (see pages 78–79).

6 Using your left hand, raise the arm above the head and hold while your other hand oils and then massages along the side of the body and into the waist. This not only feels wonderful, but it can also help relieve back and kidney ache.

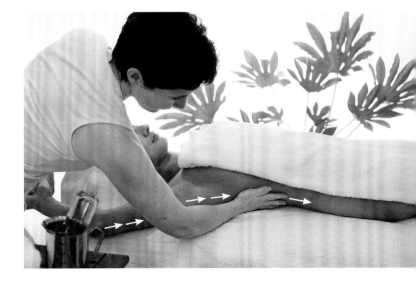

abhyanga: abdomen

This sequence focuses on small vortexes of energy called Marma points. They correspond with the seven principal chakras and are seen as meeting points along the body's energy pathways—similar in principle to acupressure points—and are an intrinsic part of Ayurvedic medicine. I have indicated the location of the Marma points where relevant.

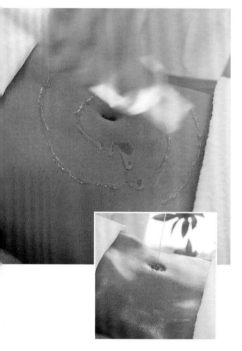

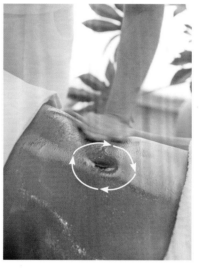

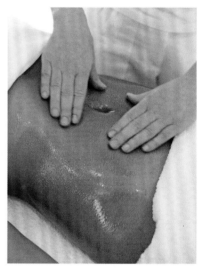

1 Cover the chest with a warm towel and uncover the abdomen. Apply warmed oil in a spiral, starting at the center and circling around the navel and outwards. End by filling the navel with oil. This not only feels good it also has a therapeutic effect on the internal organs.

2 Massage the abdomen gently with your flat palm using clockwise strokes. This further lubricates the internal organs. Nabhi abhyanga (navel massage) is an important part of Ayurvedic massage as the abdomen is regarded as the seat of spiritual and physical energy, known as the Hara.

3 Using both hands now, and leading with your thumbs, lightly massage over the navel in a straight line, using an up-and-down motion, as if lightly kneading dough. This continues the beneficial effect on the internal organs.

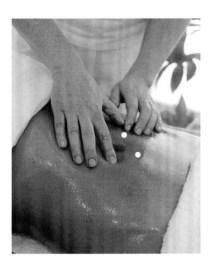 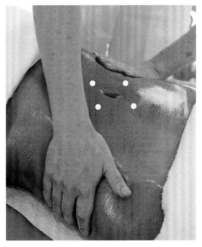 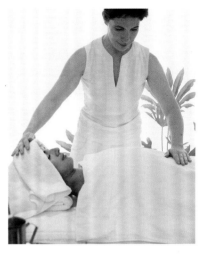

4 Using your first and second fingers, press the relevant inner Marma points, 2in (5cm) from the navel in the following positions: 12 o'clock (heart/lung), 3 o'clock (spleen/pancreas), 6 o'clock (reproductive organs/colon), and 9 o'clock (liver/gallbladder).

5 Once you have completed the Marma point massage, massage again clockwise and then add more oil to the navel area. The oil calms the Hara and oils the internal organs more deeply, giving a sense of peace and contentment.

6 Cover the recipient with a towel. Once again, place the palms of one hand on the third eye or Ajna chakra on the forehead and the other on the solar plexus chakra, Manipura. By doing this you are connecting the Hara with the third eye and, as before, this calms the spirit enough to express divine Prana in the earthly world.

MAJOR MARMA POINTS

The Ajna, or third eye chakra, is the main energy point used to balance Vata and some of its functions: mental capacity, digestion, lungs, and heart.

The Anahata, or heart chakra, is the main energy point to balance Pitta and some of its functions: general blood flow and circulation, hormones, and spiritual incentives.

The Manipura, or solar plexus chakra, is the main energy point to balance Kapha and some of its functions: kidneys, urinary system, and metabolism.

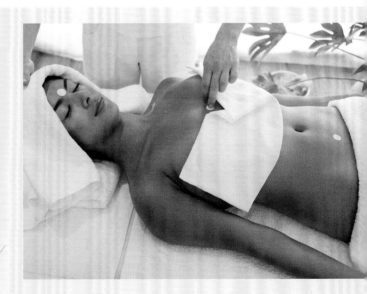

abhyanga: front of legs and feet

This sequence of massages focuses on the energy channels in the legs, easing tension and helping to combat fluid retention. It is especially beneficial for Kapha individuals, but all Dosha types will enjoy these movements.

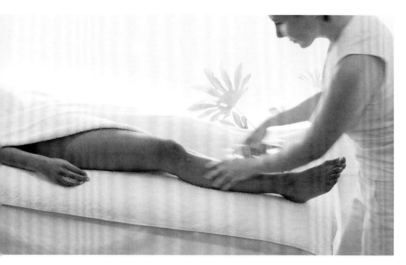

1 Uncover one leg and drape the towel discreetly over the other leg. Cover the leg with warmed oil, taking care to pour with one hand, as you spread the oil and massage with the other.

2 Rhythmically rub and lightly push the oil into the skin, counting three sets of five strokes. Use the appropriate stroke movements for the recipient's Dosha type—light and slow for Vata, medium pressure and speed for Pitta, and stimulating and fast for Kapha.

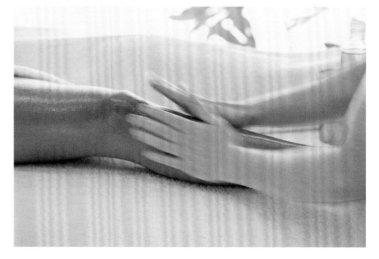

3 Now use both hands to knead the thigh. This step is especially good for the Kapha-dominant person, who may be retaining fluid in their legs or feeling generally sluggish. It can also be used for Pitta types but might feel a bit abrasive to Vata-dominant individuals.

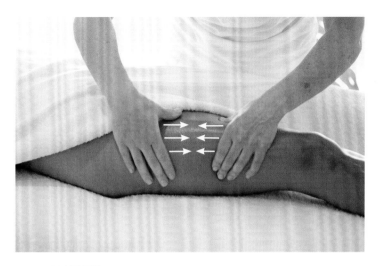

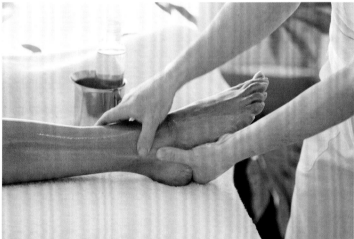

4 Hold the recipient's leg steady with one hand and then, using your thumb primarily, with fingers adding support, massage up the energy channels of the leg muscles—left, middle, right.

5 Still holding the leg with one hand, raise the leg and gently flex and extend the foot with the other hand. This helps free any energy that has been building up, ready to be released in the foot massage that follows.

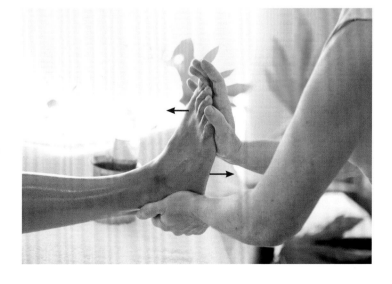

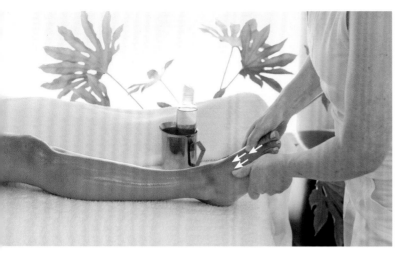

6 Now the Padabhyanga (foot massage). First, saturate the foot with oil. Supporting the foot with one hand, use your thumb to massage upwards in little nudging movements, following the channels between the bones on the top of the foot.

7 Using both hands, massage the whole of the foot, leading with the thumbs and moving from the center, outwards and downwards.

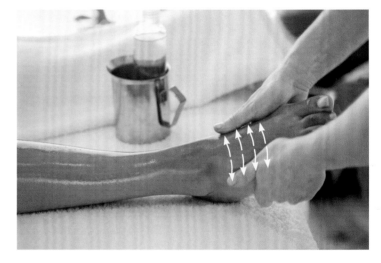

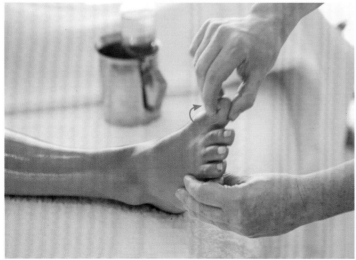

8 Using squeezing, rotating, and pressing movements, massage each toe, starting with the big toe and working along to the little toe. This relieves aching feet and also activates the many Marma energy points in the feet. Repeat the whole sequence on the other leg.

abhyanga: the back

Unlike other massage techniques, Ayurvedic massage allows the muscles to simply melt with the sensation of the hot oil and the deep lubrication it provides. I use a variety of different strokes, such as friction, percussion, heel of palm, and pull-ups, adjusting the pace and pressure to suit the recipient's dominant Dosha.

1 Make sure the oil is still warm. If need be, top up the metal container with more hot water. When you are ready to continue the massage, pull back the towel to uncover the recipient's back.

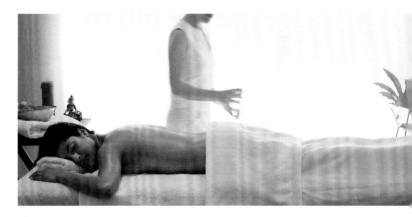

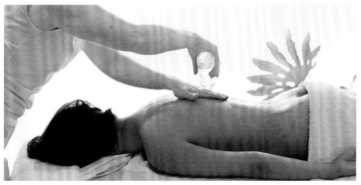

2 Standing at the head of the recipient, pour the oil over the back of your own hand as you massage, flat palm moving down the spine. Lubricate the back well; we aim to use a lot of oil in Ayurvedic massage (remember, three bottles for Vata and Pitta and two for Kapha).

3 Continue by spreading more oil and massaging down the back and around the arms, using the relevant technique according to the dominant Dosha of the recipient.

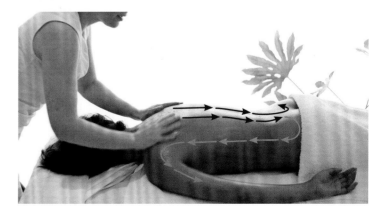

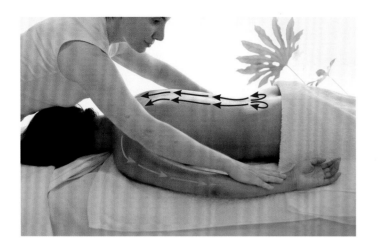

4 Start at the lower back, circle and sweep from the center of the lower back to the upper back, and continue along the arms. You could also approach this step standing at the side of the recipient (see step 5).

5 Oil the back again using the Ayurvedic method of pouring the oil through your fingers as before. Administer strokes according to the recipient's dominant Dosha, as follows:

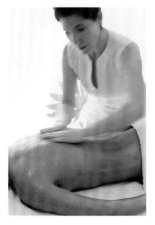

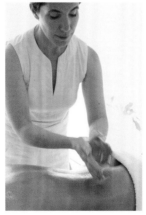

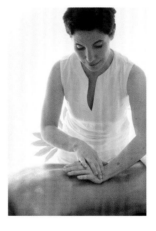

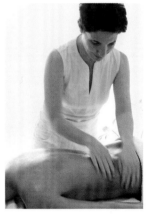

Friction
With hands side by side and palms flat, rub the back with repetitive strokes—slow for Vata, medium for Pitta, and fast for Kapha.

Percussion
Using the sides of both hands, percuss (tap repeatedly) along the back with little karate chops. This is a good stroke for Kapha- and Pitta-dominant people. Take care to avoid the spine.

Heel of palm
Use the heel of one hand to massage the back with a series of upward strokes, while pressing with the other hand to provide additional pressure. This technique is good for Pitta and Kapha types.

Pull up
Using both palms alternately, in a right then left motion, gently pull the flesh towards you. Vary the speed to suit the recipient's Dosha. This step is good for all Doshic types.

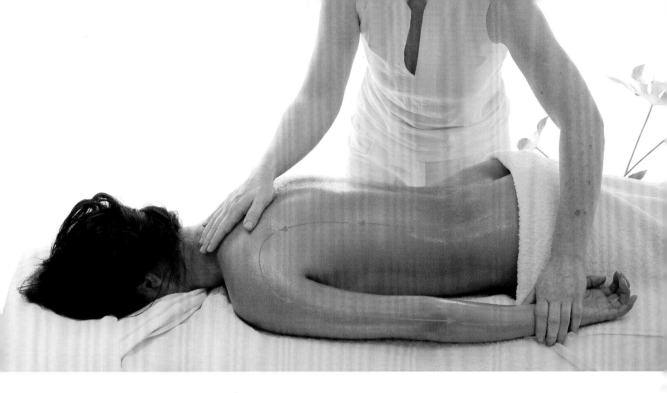

6 Administer more oil (you'll probably be surprised by just how much is absorbed!). Continue with long sweeping strokes, one hand following the other, working up the side of the spine, along the middle of the back, and around the arm. Repeat on the other side.

7 To end this sequence, cover the recipient's back and place one hand on top of the crown chakra, Adhipati, and the other on the root chakra at the base of the spine.

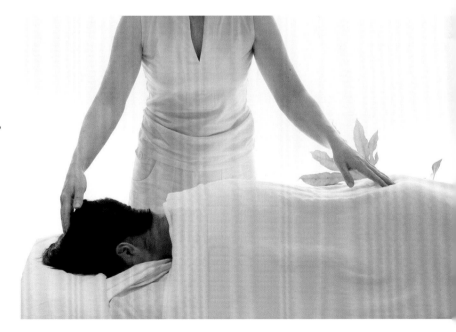

abhyanga: backs of legs

This sequence concentrates first on the legs and then on the feet to complete the Abhyanga. After you have finished the massage itself, allow plenty of time for the recipient to rest and be at one with themselves.

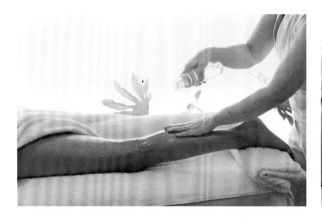

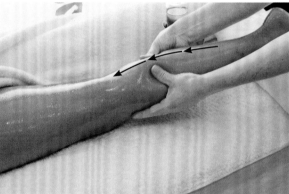

1 Move back the towel to uncover one leg and spread the oil with the flat palm. For Vata and Pitta types, make sure you saturate the whole leg, as the skin here is often dry and neglected. Use less oil for the Kapha-dominant person, as it can exacerbate their symptoms.

2 Trace the midline of the calf muscle using your hands, leading with the thumbs. Use quick, light strokes for Pitta- and Kapha-dominant people and slower strokes for Vata types.

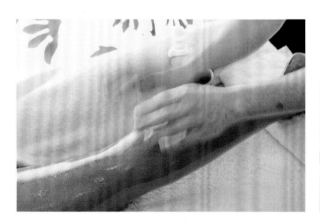

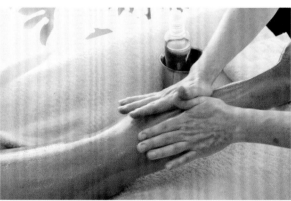

3 Using both hands side by side, tap the calf muscle rhythmically, keeping your fingers flexible. This is a really good stimulating stroke—ideal for Kapha.

4 Cross your hand at the thumb and rub using your flat palms—again, vary the speed and depth according to Doshic type. I think this technique is particularly good for Vata types as it suits a slow, light approach.

5 Complete the Abhyanga with a foot massage, using the appropriate stroke for the Dosha of the recipient, as follows: Vata—smoothing, Pitta—circling, Kapha—tapping. Now repeat the sequence on the other leg and foot.

6 Connect the crown chakra with the sacral chakra, sacrum with knees, and knees with feet. Allow the recipient to rest for 5–15 minutes before rising. They can lie either on their front, side, or back, whichever they prefer. Cover them with a warm blanket.

To finish the session, hold both feet and sound "aum," or ring Tibetan bells, as you did at the start. In this way you complete the circle, integrating the harmony of the cosmos.

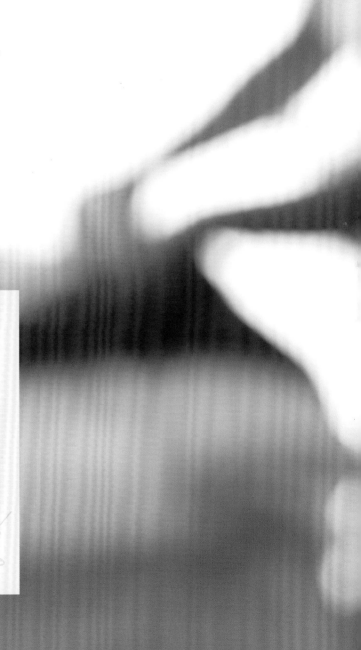

UTVARTANA DRY SKIN BRUSHING

Dry skin brushing is a very good addition to the Kapha Abhyanga when you have finished the oil massage, or it may be used as a relaxing substitute. It also makes a perfect form of self-treatment.

Dry skin brush before a hot shower in the morning if you would like to decrease Kapha. Cover the recipient with barley or chickpea flour, shaken through a baking sieve, and then dry brush the whole area with a hand-held soft skin brush.

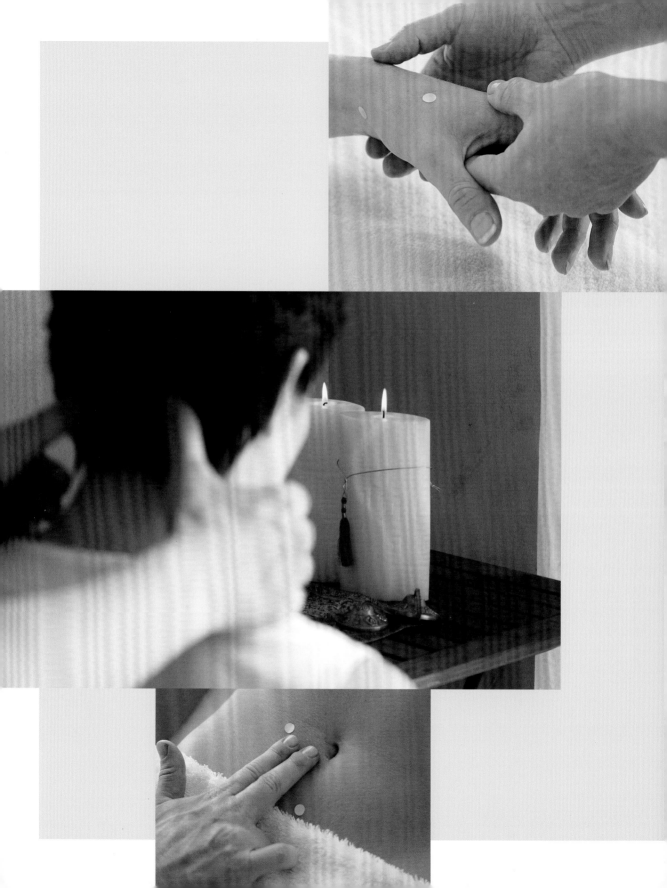

acupressure

My fascination with Traditional Chinese Medicine (TCM) began when I visited China many years ago, soon after leaving university, and has continued undiminished ever since. TCM is an ancient healing system that integrates natural therapies such as Eastern herbalism, massage, and diet into a holistic or "whole body" approach to health.

Acupressure plays an important part in TCM, both as a self-help measure and as a therapeutic aid to help others. In this section, I look at acupressure and explain how this powerful treatment system can help you maintain your physical and emotional wellbeing, easily and naturally.

what is acupressure?

Acupressure is a potent system of healing, used to treat emperors and country folk alike, which originated in China over 4,000 years ago. It is similar to acupuncture in many ways. In fact, acupressure preceded acupuncture as a form of healing. Both employ a map of trigger points—known as acupoints—that punctuate the energetic pathways or channels called Meridians. These channels pass over the surface of the body and also deep inside it. But whereas acupuncture treats acupoints with the use of needles, acupressure utilizes thumb or finger pressure.

Acupressure was originally performed by doctors whose knowledge and training were passed on from generation to generation. It offered a simple yet effective form of treatment to rural people. No additional tools were needed and so it was suited to the agrarian life of simplicity. Acupressure is part of a wider treatment system called Traditional Chinese Medicine (TCM). This has its origins in an ancient and naturalistic Chinese philosophy called Taoism. TCM integrates the natural elements into a belief structure that reflects, in its larger form, the macrocosm of the cosmos and, in its smaller form, the microcosm of the human being.

Traditional Chinese Medicine is based on a belief that man does not exist in isolation but is an intricate part of the cosmos. The cosmos is ruled

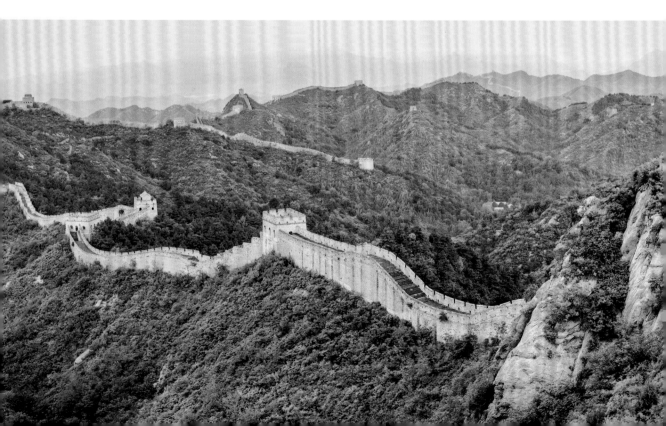

YIN AND YANG

Yin and Yang are equal, integral parts of the universe and life. The Yin/Yang symbol represents all universal life in harmony. Chinese medicine aims to achieve balance between these forces of nature, environment, and man himself.

Yin organs	Yang organs
Liver	Gall Bladder
Heart	Small Intestine
Spleen	Stomach
Lungs	Large Intestine
Kidneys	Urinary Bladder

Yin	Yang
Feminine	Masculine
Night	Day
Internal	External
Cool	Warm
Intuitive	Rational
Serene	Excited
Receptive	Expressive
Light	Dark
Passive	Active

by two opposing but mutually dependent forces— Yin and Yang (see right). True health is possible only when one is in harmony with the environment, community, and season, and when mind and body are one. This is achieved by keeping Yin and Yang in balance. So, if we are in generally good physical health but often feel angry and irritable, we are not in harmony.

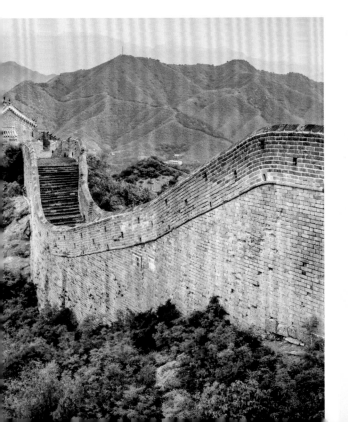

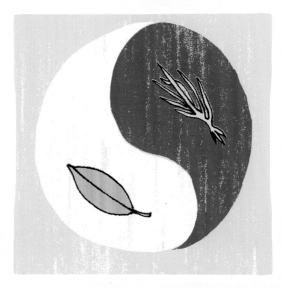

the benefits of acupressure

Acupressure can be used to calm or stimulate mind and body and so restore the individual to natural stasis and balance—physically, emotionally, and spiritually. We naturally massage our temples when we have a headache or rub our muscles to ease aches and pains. When we do this we are instinctively using acupressure principles by applying pressure and friction to key points in order to restore calm to the body.

Acupressure is not just a great pain reliever but is also used to control the flow of energy, called Chi (or Qi), that passes through the Meridians, thereby bringing about a state of equilibrium of mind and body. The body has hundreds of acupoints. They are like little energetic vortexes that allow easy access to the Meridians. They can be stimulating or sedating, depending on how pressure is applied to them, which is determined by the needs of the recipient at that particular moment. Acupressure can boost the flow of Chi energy to relieve tiredness or weakness, or ease the flow to calm overactive conditions. It can balance the hormones, support fertility and potency, and help the recipient reconnect with their deepest self.

Don't be misled by the fact that acupoints are so easy to access and use. These points are very powerful, so always approach them with respect and caution, as well as a good measure of confidence, as I guide you on this ancient Chinese journey of healing.

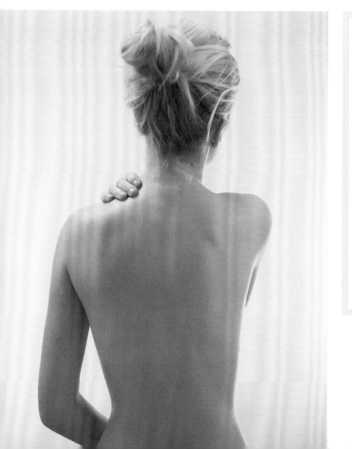

CAUTION

Acupressure is safe for treating minor ailments such as a headache and lower back pain but should not take the place of professional advice. Contact a qualified acupuncturist or acupressure practitioner for professional treatment. Never use acupressure on the elderly, or anyone who is pregnant, has high blood pressure, or is ill. Do not use implements to stimulate the acupoints. Acupuncture, and any use of needles, should only be performed by trained and licensed acupuncturists.

emotional health and acupressure

According to Traditional Chinese Medicine, emotions originate in particular organs and can affect overall health. These organs are not just physical structures but systems with wide-ranging influences on the body. In this way emotion and bodily organ are closely linked.

If the organ is out of balance or the emotion is overloaded, one will have an effect on the other. For example, an extended period of kidney problems may make someone fearful or lack self-esteem. If they have suffered a bereavement and have grieved for a long time, they may find their lung energy becomes depleted, leading to colds and flu. Even a positive emotion such as joy can cause an imbalance, leading to manic behavior. In Taoist tradition, a calm observation of one's emotions is the foundation stone for a long and healthy life. TCM treats both physical and emotional state simultaneously.

For Westerners, who are not used to regarding their emotions in this way, I would advocate trying not to dwell too much on any one emotion. Be completely in the moment. Feel your emotions deeply—and then let them go. Interestingly, modern scientific research shows that repeated anger can

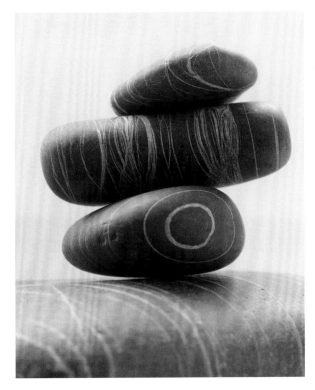

exaggerate the production of brain chemicals called neuropeptides. If you have felt anger for a long period it can lead to a pattern of neural pathways and neuropeptide release that can become a negative cycle.

ACUPRESSURE AND THE EMOTIONS

organ	associated emotion	acupoint
Liver	Anger, frustration, and irritability	Liv–2
Heart	Joy, excessive joy, and excitement	Ht–5
Spleen	Worry, over-thinking, and circular thought	Sp–6
Lungs	Grief, remorse, and depression	Lu–1
Kidney	Fear, shock, and lack of confidence	Ki–6
Small Intestine	Indecision and lack of direction	Si–3

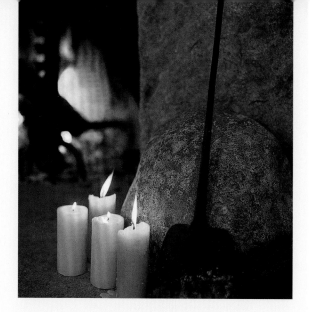

working with acupoints

Acupoints allow the therapist to influence the flow of Chi energy. The Chinese often liken Chi to the flow of water, sometimes languidly collecting in pools, at other times energetically tumbling over rocks.

Each acupoint intersects with the flow of Chi at a particular location along one of the Meridian pathways and so is uniquely placed to control the Chi—either calming an over-energetic flow, or stimulating a sluggish one. In Traditional Chinese Medicine the acupoints have poetic names reflecting their function, such as "Yang Pool," but in the West we use abbreviations that reflect the organ system influenced and the position on the Meridian. See illustrations (right) for locations of the acupoints and the box (below right) for key to abbreviations.

ORGANS, SEASONS, ELEMENTS, AND ENERGY

The five principal organs correspond to the five elements of Traditional Chinese Medicine: Heart—Fire, Lung—Metal, Spleen—Earth, Liver—Wood, and Kidney—Water. In addition, four of these elements relate to the seasons: Fire—Summer, Metal—Autumn, Water—Winter, and Wood—Spring. The seasons all have a direct impact on the fifth element—Earth. In this way, Chinese medicine draws together all aspects of nature, the elements, the seasons, and bodily systems into one unifying theory.

These five organ systems have their own Meridians or energy pathways plus associated acupoints, as do all the other organ systems. In addition, practitioners of Chinese medicine envisage other pathways in the body, for which there is no comparable organ in Western medicine. These act as "overflow" channels when there is an overabundance of Chi energy. These channels, too, have their associated acupoints. Only a few of these additional channels are regularly used in Chinese medicine. They are the Conception Vessel (CV), the Triple Burner (TB), and the Governor Vessel (GV).

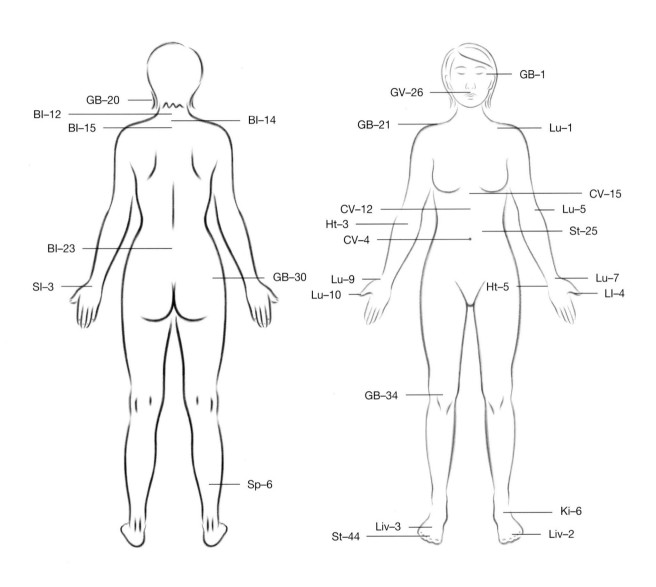

GB–20
Bl–12
Bl–15
Bl–14
Bl–23
GB–30
SI–3
Sp–6

GB–1
GV–26
GB–21
Lu–1
CV–15
CV–12
Lu–5
Ht–3
St–25
CV–4
Lu–9
Lu–7
Lu–10
LI–4
Ht–5
GB–34
Ki–6
Liv–3
Liv–2
St–44

KEY TO ACUPOINTS

Bl	Bladder	Ht	Heart	Lu	Lungs
CV	Conception Vessel	Ki	Kidney	SI	Small Intestine
GB	Gall Bladder	LI	Large Intestine	Sp	Spleen
GV	Governing Vessel	Liv	Liver	St	Stomach

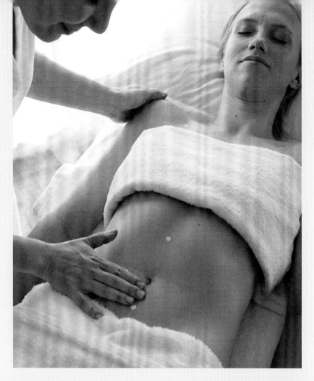

Two important acupoints on the abdomen help maintain emotional balance. CV–12, located four finger widths above the navel, promotes a sense of wellbeing. CV–4, located four finger widths below the navel, reduces mental anguish.

acupressure for health

Acupressure is perfect for self-massage or can be used to treat a friend for a minor ailment. For example, activating GV–26, in the indentation in the middle of the upper lip, relieves facial tension. Activating LI–4, in the web of skin between thumb and first finger, relieves facial pain, blocked sinuses, and headache.

The acupressure sequence I am sharing with you can be used as an oil-free massage—self-contained and powerful, or within the massage on the move sequences, or can make a perfect addition to the simple healing massage.

I tend to use acupressure as part of my simple healing massage. If, for example, the recipient has a cold and they have come for a massage I will use the acupressure points during the massage to help relieve the symptoms. This makes the simple healing massage a more powerful treatment.

During the winter I activate the Chi-boosting points of the kidneys, heart, and lungs. This strengthens the defensive Chi energy and keeps the immunity strong to protect against the chills of the winter, as well as other people's germs!

acupressure techniques

The acupoints and massage techniques here can be integrated into oil-massage sequences, used in healing sessions, or used as part of a simple dry massage on the move.

Before applying acupressure techniques on others, find some accessible acupoints on yourself. Acupoints are often located in little dips or depressions, for example between the finger or toe bones, or at the base of the skull. You will know when you have located an acupoint because you will feel a slight tingling sensation. As the body is symmetrical, many acupoints are in pairs on each side of the body and can often be stimulated at the same time.

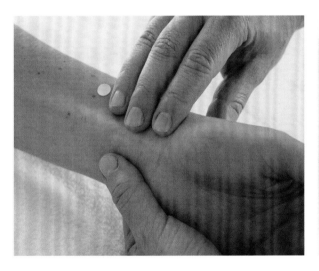

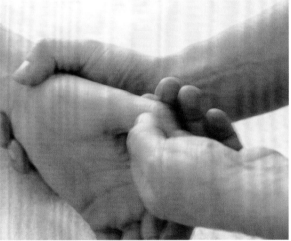

1 Point location

To identify the locations of the acupoints, I use a Chinese measurement called a "cun," based on finger widths. This example shows a position three finger widths up from the wrist. Always feel for the little dip or point of connection that is the acupressure point.

2 Thumb-roll activation

For extra pressure, you can activate acupoints using the "thumb-roll" method. Place the pad of your thumb on the acupoint and apply a little pressure to press in a circular movement—clockwise to relax or sedate and counterclockwise to stimulate or tonify.

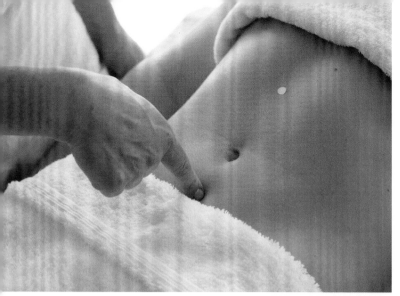

3 The power index finger

Use your first finger to stimulate the acupressure point by applying controlled, cautious pressure. As you do, imagine the golden light of healing emanating from your finger to stimulate the point. Make sure your nails are short for this.

4 Fingertip rotation

In this movement you use your first finger or your second finger—if that is stronger—to activate the point in a circular motion, applying slight pressure.

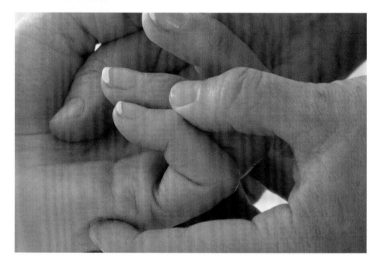

HOW TO ACTIVATE AN ACUPOINT

Begin by locating the point, then using either your thumb or finger, feel for the dip that the point naturally has—sometimes this is very subtle, and other times more obvious. Once you have located the point, apply a gentle pressure at first. Then press in to the acupoint, using a slight rotating and pressing action—this will activate the Chi, or energy of the acupoint, and the Meridian it relates to.

If you are using acupressure on someone else, do so with great care (see the cautionary notes on page 101). Let your recipient know from the start that you will stop at any point, should they ask you to. Always closely observe your recipient's expression and body language to monitor how they are experiencing your touch and adjust the pressure accordingly.

5 Double-thumb power

You can use both thumbs simultaneously for greater effect. Use circular motions to activate and clear the acupoints and hold the thumbs in position to stimulate and tonify.

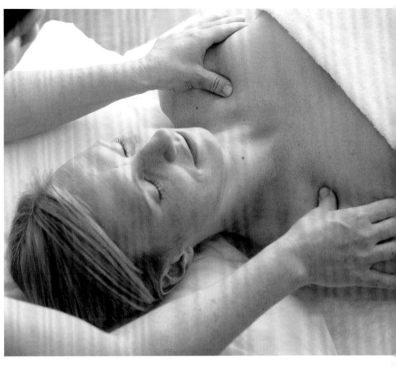

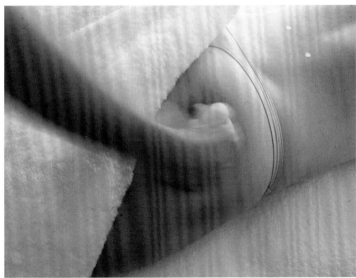

6 Fist rotation

Make fists and rotate with pressure into this deep point. Either alternate the action of each fist or do this technique simultaneously with both fists.

to ease headaches and cold symptoms and to lift your spirits

The acupoints on the hands and arms intersect with Meridian pathways that have a strong influence on the face and chest. Because of this they are particularly effective at alleviating cold and flu symptoms, such as facial tension and pain, blocked sinuses, chesty cough, and general fatigue and lethargy. Other acupoints shown here can lift mood and promote restful sleep. As the hands and arms are so easily accessible, you can try these techniques on yourself, at home or at work, or even on the move.

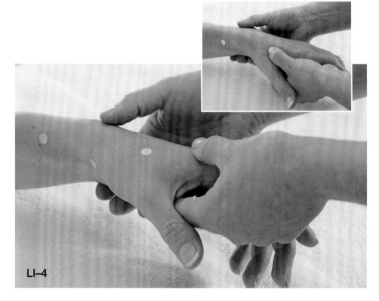

LI–4 is located at the central point in the web between the thumb and first finger. This is a powerful point to alleviate headaches especially at the front of the head and ease facial pain, toothache, and tension in the jaw. It also alleviates blocked sinuses, sneezing, coughs, and colds, aids mental clarity, and eases feelings of worry and anxiety.

LI–4

Lu–5

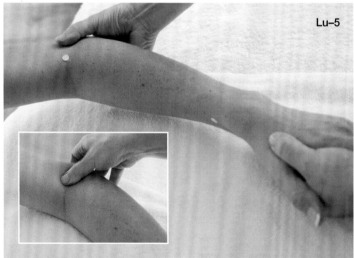

Lu–5 is located in the hollow of the elbow, on the outer (lateral) border of the tendon. This point alleviates coughs and bronchitis with yellow/white mucus, it relieves pain in the elbow and forearm and it helps ease feelings of loss.

Lu–7 is located three finger widths above the wrist, with palm side up. This is a powerful point for coughs and colds. It promotes sweating and eases blocked sinuses, loss of smell, and sneezing. This point also reduces oedema and fluid retention.

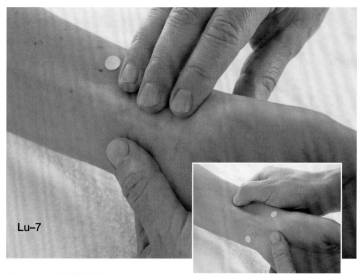

Lu–7

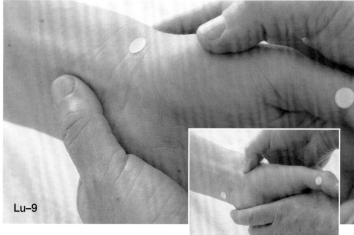

Lu–9

Lu–9 is located at the wrist bone, palm side up. This point strengthens lung Chi to aid a weak voice and shallow breathing. It dissipates lethargy and promotes blood circulation. It also strengthens lung Yin to clear phlegm from the lungs and alleviates symptoms such as dry cough and feeling hot or thirsty all the time.

CAUTION

Acupressure is a very safe therapy to use for young and old alike. Nevertheless, it is always wise to take simple precautions if there is a risk of causing harm, no matter how slight.

• Never apply acupressure to another person or yourself if you have been drinking alcohol or feel faint.

• Work around cuts, wounds, bruises, or varicose veins and never apply acupressure directly to these areas.

• Stop immediately if the recipient feels unwell or faint. Consult a professional.

• Do not perform acupressure during pregnancy.

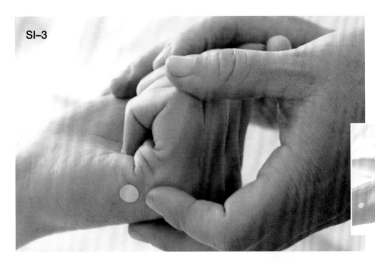

SI-3

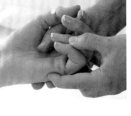

SI-3 is located on the fold that appears when the hand makes a fist. This point eases vertigo, neck stiffness and headaches, relaxes muscles and tendons of the upper back, clears the mind, and strengthens judgment.

Ht-3 is located in the indentation on the inside of the elbow fold, next to the tendon. This point eases depression and uplifts the spirit, alleviates insomnia, and calms angst-filled dreams.

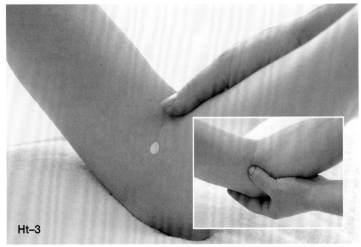

Ht-3

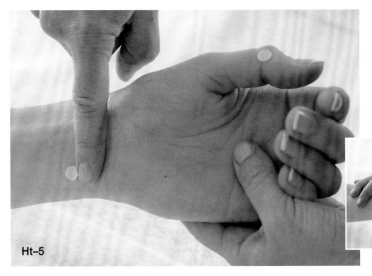

Ht-5

Ht-5 is located one finger width up on the wrist and on the inside of the wrist tendon. This point eases mild palpitations (but do not use in serious cases), alleviates stage fright, and promotes a feeling of joy and confidence.

to help ease migraine and abdominal pain and to calm irritability

The acupoints on the legs and feet intersect the Liver, Gall Bladder, Spleen, and Stomach Meridians and have a major influence on the abdomen. They can alleviate digestive upsets, such as indigestion, nausea, abdominal pain, and bloating (common symptoms in irritable bowel syndrome), and menstrual problems.

GB–34 is located just below the kneecap and at the side of the knee. This point is good for relieving IBS symptoms, bloating, and abdominal pain. It alleviates nausea, indigestion, and menstrual congestion and strengthens the legs.

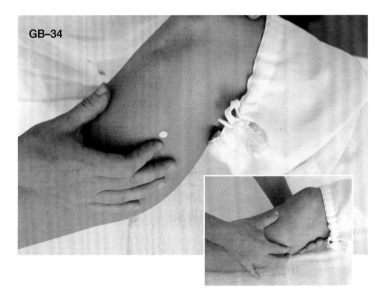

GB–34

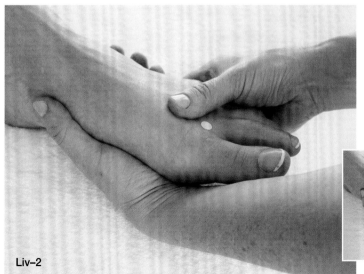

Liv–2

Liv–2 is located between the big toe and the second toe. This point eases headaches, red eyes, and insomnia. It alleviates dizziness and vertigo and may be useful in calming heavy menstrual flow. It also subdues feelings of anger and frustration.

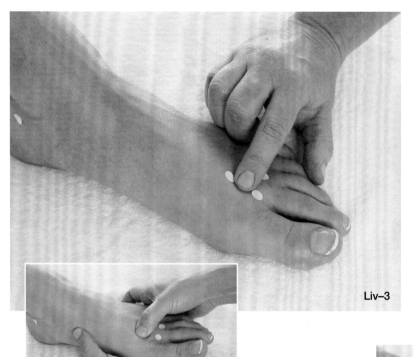

Liv–3 is one finger width up from Liv–2 (see page 103). This point eases constriction in the abdomen and head and alleviates symptoms of migraine. It calms the mind, eases tension, frustration, and irritability, and relieves depression.

Liv–3

Sp–6 is four finger widths above the ankle bone. This point alleviates menstrual cramps, especially when clotting is present. It eases premenstrual syndrome and regulates menstruation. It also relieves frustration and tension, and eases hot flushes and dry mouth at night.

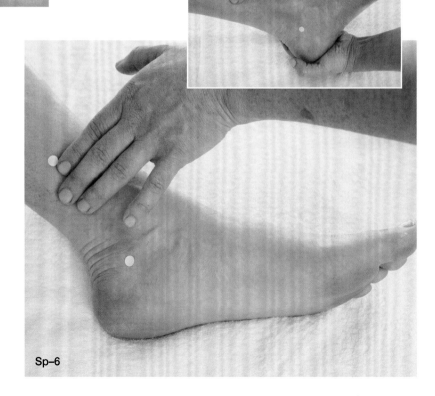

Sp–6

St–44 is located in the hollow between the second and third toe bones, just above the toes. This point eases feelings of fullness or pain in the stomach, alleviates heartburn, calms nosebleeds, bleeding gums and toothache, and improves focus and judgment.

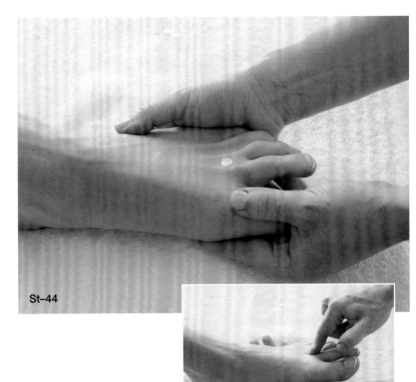

St–44

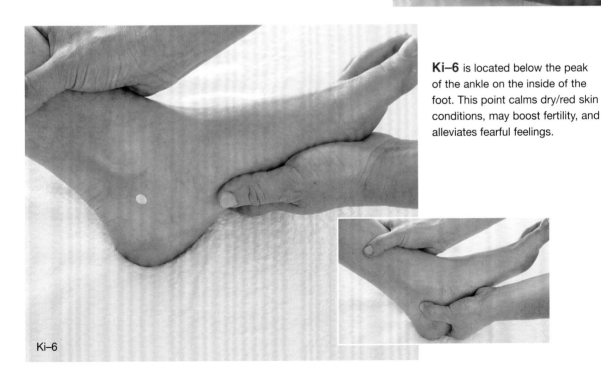

Ki–6

Ki–6 is located below the peak of the ankle on the inside of the foot. This point calms dry/red skin conditions, may boost fertility, and alleviates fearful feelings.

to ease digestive disorder, alleviate coughs, and aid tranquility

The link between our emotional state and chest and abdominal symptoms is well known. When we are nervous or anxious, we feel "butterflies" or tightening in the stomach, and our breathing can become rapid and shallow. No surprise, then, that stimulating acupoints on the chest and abdomen can dramatically affect our mood, relieving apprehension, and promoting confidence and general feelings of wellbeing.

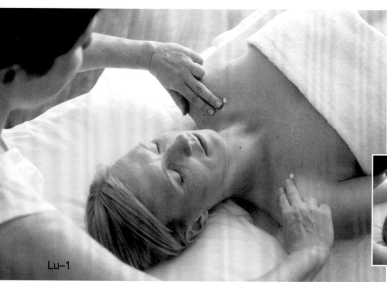

Lu–1 is located two finger widths below the point where the clavicle meets the shoulder. This point eases coughs and a build-up of phlegm in the lungs. It calms feelings of grief or regret, alleviates constriction in the chest area, and promotes the confidence to let go of the past.

Lu–1

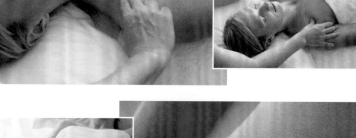

St–25 is located two finger widths to the side of the navel. This point eases abdominal swelling and constipation. It relieves burning pain and diarrhea and calms manic behavior.

St–25

CV–4 is located in the center of the abdomen, four finger widths below the navel. This point strengthens the kidneys, tonifies the uterus, and is purported to boost fertility. It also reduces mental anguish.

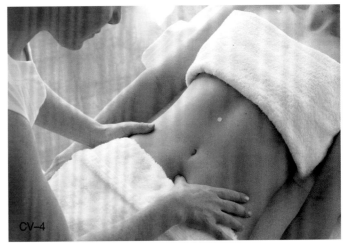

CV–4

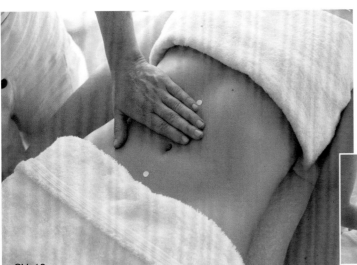

CV–12

CV–12 is located four finger widths above the navel. This point strengthens the stomach, especially if there is digestive weakness, improves appetite, and promotes a sense of wellbeing.

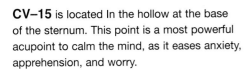

CV–15 is located In the hollow at the base of the sternum. This point is a most powerful acupoint to calm the mind, as it eases anxiety, apprehension, and worry.

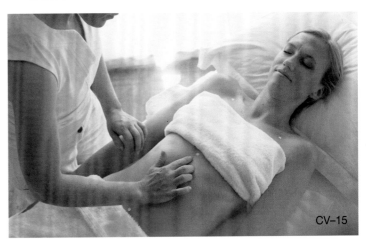

CV–15

to ease eye and ear problems and reduce over-thinking

Many common ills are a consequence of our modern lifestyle and working practices. Sitting for long periods, staring at a computer or television screen, or working in a noisy environment can lead to sore eyes, muscle aches and stiffness, tension, and headache. After extended periods of this sort of treatment, we can become generally run down and therefore at greater risk of common complaints such as colds, coughs, and flu. The acupoints on these pages can alleviate many of these symptoms and also strengthen the body's resistance to infection. You can apply them on their own or incorporate them into a healing massage.

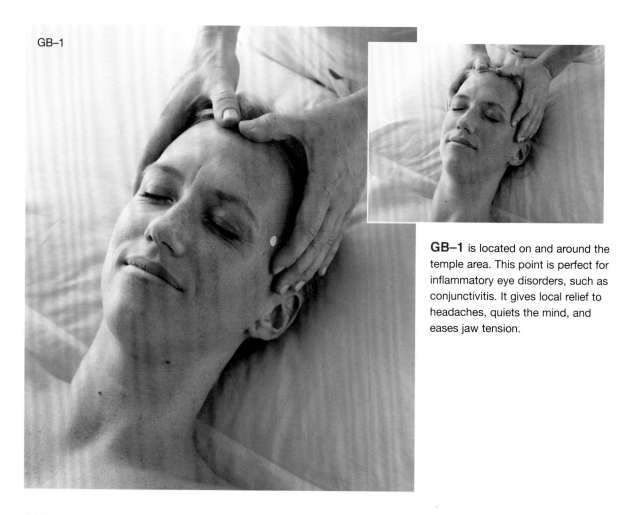

GB–1

GB–1 is located on and around the temple area. This point is perfect for inflammatory eye disorders, such as conjunctivitis. It gives local relief to headaches, quiets the mind, and eases jaw tension.

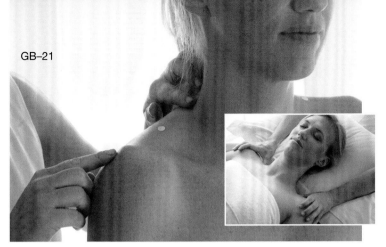

GB–21

GB–21 is located in little dips in the middle of the tops of the shoulders. This is the main point to ease muscular tension in the neck and shoulders. It promotes the flow of milk in a nursing mother.

GV–26 is located in the middle of the indentation in the upper lip. This is the main point to clear any blemishes, ease facial tension in general, and boost a radiant complexion.

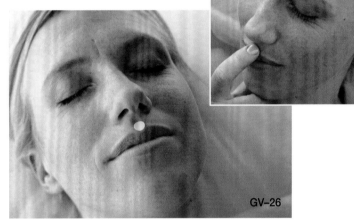

GV–26

GB–20

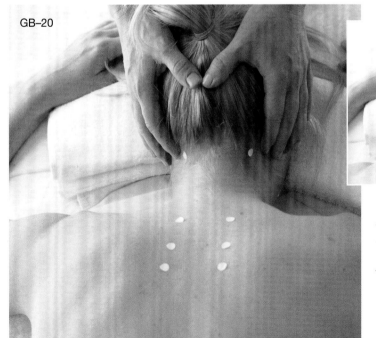

GB–20 is located in the hollows of the occiput on either side of the base of the skull. This point eases neck stiffness, headache, and earache due to colds or flu. It also alleviates dizziness, and eye and ear problems.

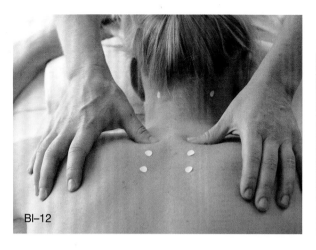

BI–12

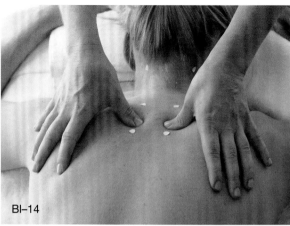

BI–14

BI–12 is located between the second and third thoracic vertebrae one and a half finger widths on either side of the spinal process. This point alleviates symptoms of cold and flu—useful if you get chilled in order to prevent a cold developing—and strengthens the lungs.

BI–14 is located between the fourth and fifth thoracic vertebrae and one and a half finger widths on either side. This point eases mental anguish and uplifts the spirit. It alleviates mild palpitations (but do not use in serious cases) and calms dental pain.

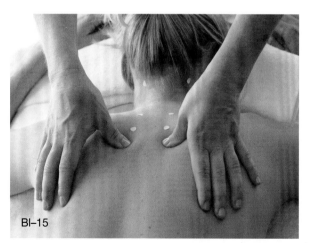

BI–15

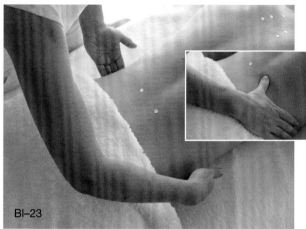

BI–23

BI–15 is located between the fifth and sixth vertebrae, one and a half finger widths either side of the spinal process. This point relieves feelings of constriction in the chest, eases insomnia, anxiety, and restlessness, and enhances memory and concentration.

BI–23 is located between the second and third lumbar vertebrae and one and a half finger widths on either side. This point relieves chronic back pain, strengthens the whole system, eases fear, and empowers the will.

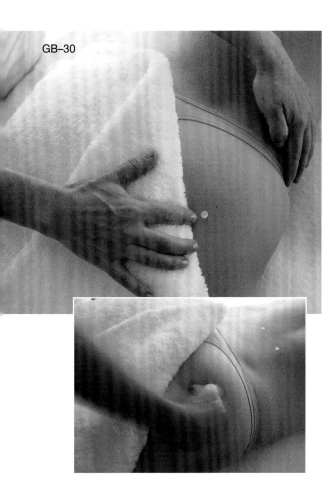

GB–30

GB–30 is located in the hollow of the buttocks on both sides. This point promotes circulation in the legs and hips, strengthens the waist and thighs, alleviates genital and anal problems or itching, and tonifies the Chi of the entire body.

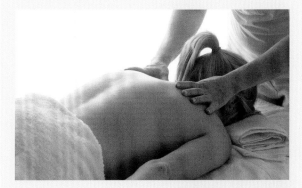

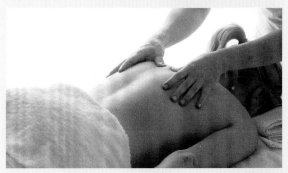

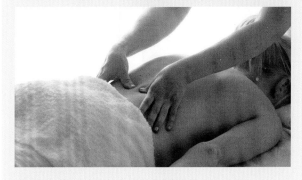

WORKING DOWN THE BACK

The paired acupoints BI–12, BI–14, and BI–15 are located on either side of the upper thoracic vertebrae. They intersect the Bladder Meridians that run in parallel on either side of the spine from the head to the bottom of the legs. This region is strongly associated with the chest and so has an important role in strengthening the respiratory tract and preventing coughs and colds, as well as calming the spirit.

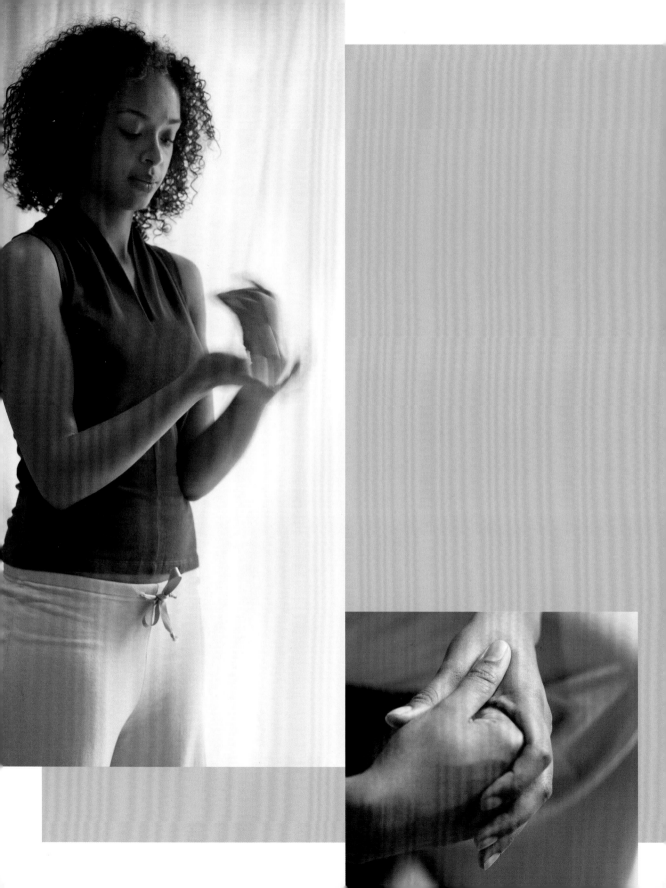

massage on the move

It is most often while traveling or having a stressful day that we feel physical and emotional tension building. These techniques—all tried-and-tested stress soothers—promote relaxation and revitalize the whole system. Whether you're at your desk, on the train, or standing in a queue, you can dip into these sequences for an instant energy boost, to calm anxiety, or to treat specific ailments, such as headache or muscle stiffness. Each routine takes no longer than five minutes, so you'll always find the time to treat yourself. It's the next best thing to having a personal masseuse with you at all times.

invigorating neck and face massage

Whenever I am feeling tired and in need of an energy boost, I use this great revitalizing sequence for my neck and face. It can help relieve neck tension, headaches, eye strain, and joint stiffness, and of course relaxes the facial muscles. As we live in a culture in which our true feelings must sometimes remain hidden, the face often becomes taut with stored stress. This sequence helps dissolve any residual tension left by the silent mask we may wear for others.

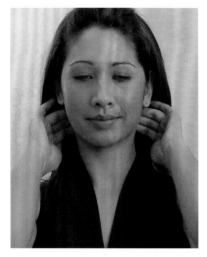 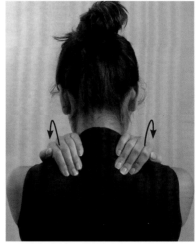 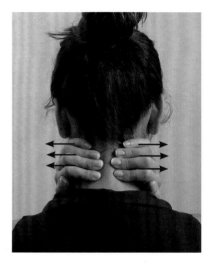

1 Allow your hands to cup the back of your neck, with the thumbs passive as supports. Let the fingertips of your first three fingers fall into the groove alongside the cervical vertebrae, or spinal bones, of your neck. Massage this area in circular movements— this can be so instantly relieving. A personal favorite of mine.

2 Begin at the top of the trapezium, the triangle of muscle at the base of the neck, and press and pull your fingers away and towards the front of your body and face. Repeat this three times and then return—a fingertip higher each time, steadily moving upwards. This is a perfect move between meetings or after a long session at the computer. I recommend a break after 45 minutes.

3 Using your fingertips, press and gently pull behind your neck. I usually move slowly upwards in five movements, with the last set of motions in the occipital ridge—the dents where the neck meets the skull. Start at the tops of the shoulders where they meet the neck and gradually move upwards. Repeat this sequence in sets of three, 10 times. It feels so natural.

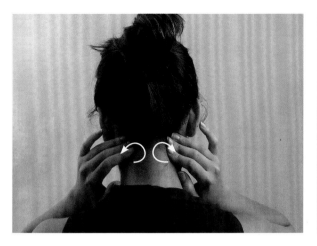

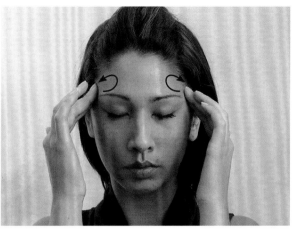

4 Allow your fingertips to rest in the occipital ridge and rotate your fingers with pressure in circular motions, alternating right then left. You will feel the tight areas here. Do this in a sequence of ten and repeat three times. This is quite a bit quicker—count "one and two and three and four" and so on.

5 Place your fingertips at your temples, repeating the circular movements used at the occipital ridge, alternating right and left. This is a powerful move to relieve tension headaches and eyestrain. Perfect if you have a headache due to over-thinking, looking at a screen for too long, or listening to incessant chatter.

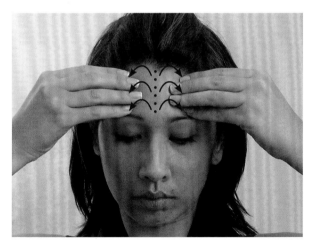

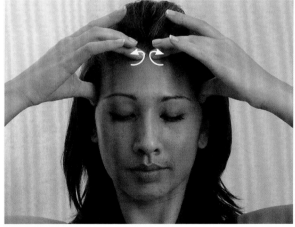

6 Allow your fingertips to meet in the center of the forehead with the thumbs resting in the temples. Again, alternate half-circle movements with your fingertips, moving from the center of your forehead to your temples. Repeat this three times. This is good for alleviating the kind of headache you may get when feeling really tired.

7 Return a fingertip higher and repeat this movement, culminating in massage along your hairline. Allow this circular sequence to follow your hairline round to the back of your neck. This step really helps relieve any tension that may have accumulated in the scalp.

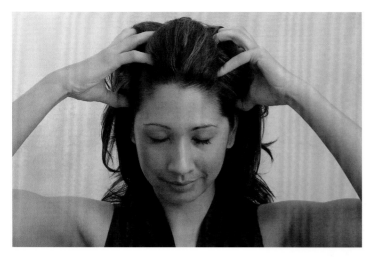

8 With all your fingers curled and your fingertips resting on your skin, as if playing the piano, let your fingers meet and make circular motions away from each hand around the crown of the head. Repeat this all over your head.

9 Place your thumbs facing upwards in the dent where your eye socket meets the eyebrow, with your first finger above your eyebrow providing support. Press with your thumbs along the underneath of the brow bone, culminating in pressing the temples, then press with your first finger along the top of the eyebrows, finishing at the temples. Repeat this sequence eight times.

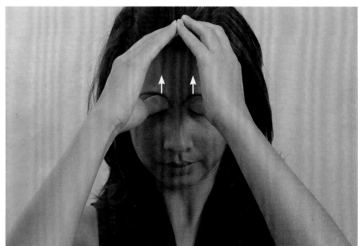

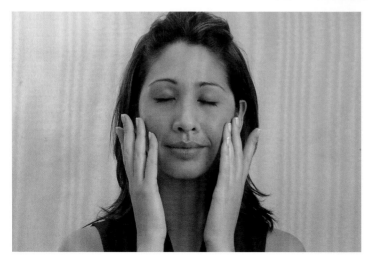

10 Lightly tap your face with open palms, your fingertips gently touching your face like the gentle flapping of butterfly wings. Concentrate this lovely movement around the jaw, too, for several moments. This can be a great radiance enhancer and complexion booster, stimulating the circulation in the face. Better than a face pack.

hand massage

Repetitive manual work such as using a computer or doing household chores can leave your hands feeling tired and aching. This revitalizing hand massage not only eases stiff, sore muscles and joints, it also activates acupoints to relieve stress and restore general wellbeing.

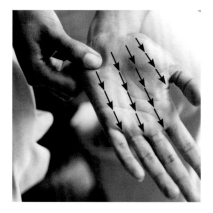

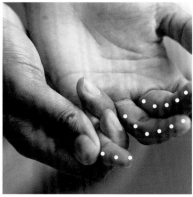

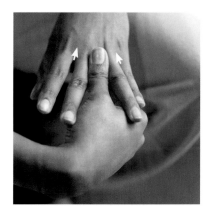

1 Using the thumb of your right hand, apply pressure as you trace the lines from your left wrist up your palm, moving an imaginary space left each time. Repeat this three times.

2 Rub each finger of your left hand between the thumb and first finger of your right hand, from the bottom of the finger up to the tip. In reflexology, the tips of the finger relate to the sinus points, so much more than just massaging the fingers.

3 Now pull gently between each finger web space. These are the reflex points for the lymphatic glands and so these movements stimulate the immune system as well as relax your fingers and hands. This is something I do whenever I feel a cold may be brewing.

4 Press into the triangular web space between your first finger and thumb. This is the acupoint LI–4, which is perfect for easing headaches and enhancing a general sense of wellbeing. This point is a potent pain reliever for the facial area.
CAUTION: Contra-indicated in pregnancy.

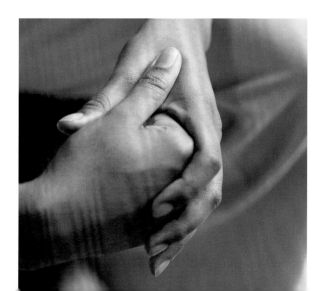

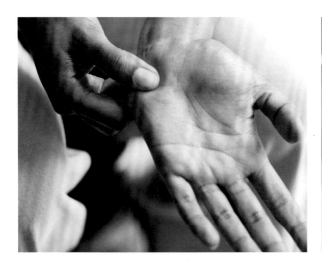

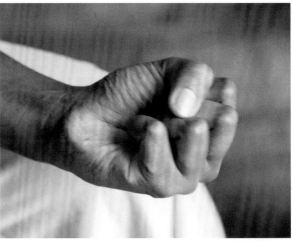

5 Now thumb roll the heel of the hand. This is a hand reflexology point that releases stress in the back. It also feels so liberating to massage the heel of the palm. I find my clients usually let out a blissful sigh when I get to this part.

6 Next, open and close the hand being massaged ten times rapidly—make a tight fist as shown, then release. This relaxes and strengthens the hand. I often use this step as a warm-up to a day of massage.

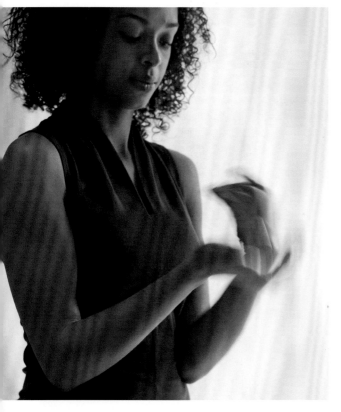

7 Flap your hands towards you gently for a count of 20. This relaxes the wrists. When I was learning to play the *djembe*, a West African hand drum, my teacher, Henri, used this movement as a warm-up exercise before class. He called it giving yourself "fresh air." We all hold a lot of stress in our wrists, a very small area considering its physically intricate nature. This is a really good move to relieve tension and keep the wrists supple—perfect after a day's work at the computer or after a session of domestic chores.

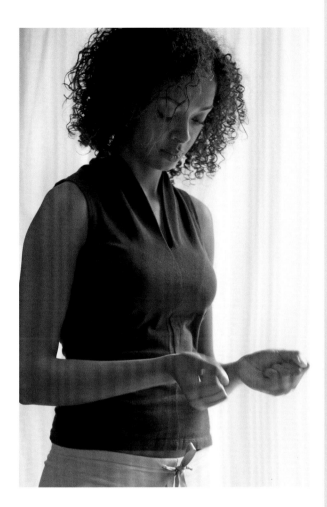

8 Rotate your wrists, first outwards and then inwards six times. Again, this helps to relieve tension in the wrists, aids strength, and maintains flexibility.

GETTING A GOOD BACK STRETCH

If there is room to lie down completely, try this great simple back stretch. Sybil Grunberg, a cranial osteopath, who I have been going to for years, shared this exercise with me. It is brilliant for releasing your lower back after you have been traveling in cramped conditions, such as a long-haul flight, or at any time.

1 Lie on the floor completely flat and bring one knee up slowly to your chest. Now slowly and gently pull it towards you. Then return your leg to a neutral lying position.

2 Repeat with the other leg—knee to chest and then back down to a neutral lying position.

3 Gently bring both knees up to your chest. Allow them to fall against you rather than pull them to you. Enjoy the gentle stretch in your lower back. Return your legs to the neutral lying position.

4 Repeat this sequence ten times.

5 Finally, kneel on the floor and gently lower your head and upper body to the floor, arms by your side until your forehead is resting on a rug or a blanket. Take deep, even breaths and feel yourself sink into the floor and your lower back and shoulders open and release. This is the "child pose," a Hatha Yoga pose that is great for releasing the whole back and quietening an overactive mind.

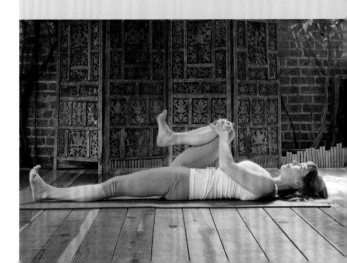

standing self-massage

This sequence is great for relieving tension and easing tired and aching muscles. It includes a Qi gong technique, beating "heaven's drum" or, as I call it, drum rolling. Simply make fists and gently tap your body as though drumming. So easy and so effective.

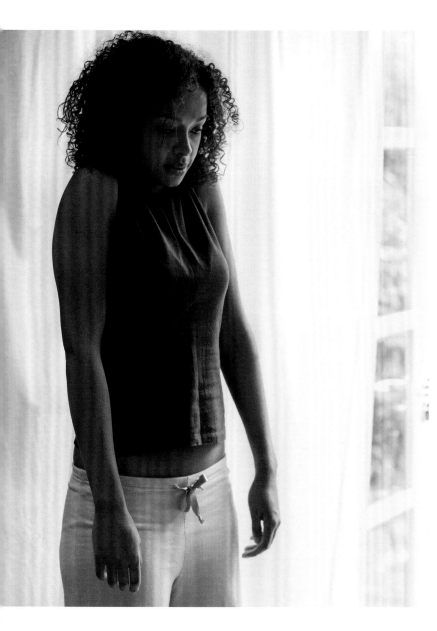

1 Begin with simple stretches—interlace fingers and raise your arms above your head—feel the gentle pull, then release. Do this to a count of eight. Repeat with hands clasped in front of you at chest height, again for a count of eight, breathing naturally. Waft your hands out to your sides, then clasp them behind you and raise them upwards behind you. Have a gentle stretch to release the trapezium muscle. Repeat this whole step in cycles of five.

2 Raise your shoulders to your ears gently and then lower them again. This, too, releases the trapezium muscle and is a perfect way to get quick relief after spending too long sitting in one position, for example when working at the computer. Do this five times.

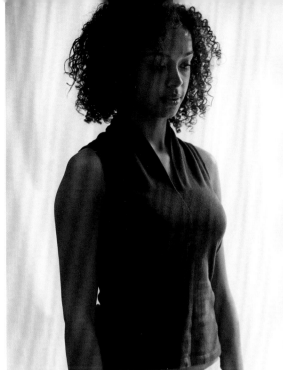

3 Stand tall. Imagine that a balloon on a string is attached to your spine and gently pulling you up yet your feet feel grounded on the earth. Imagine all your energy draining down your spine, clearing away through the soles of your feet and into the depths of the earth. Take ten slow, even breaths and visualize the release. Repeat ten times.

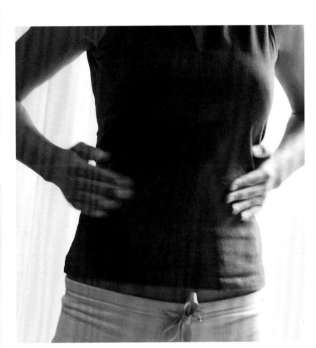

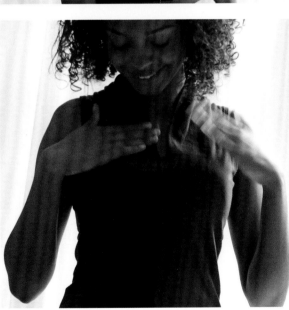

5 Pat yourself gently and rhythmically around your ribcage to the front; this helps to re-enliven the diaphragm. Follow the line from the breastbone, where the ribs meet, to the softer part of the stomach. Continue patting between the breasts onto your chest.

4 Stand with feet hip-width apart. Breathe evenly. Pat yourself across your upper chest. Keep patting up to the tops of your shoulders. This simple yet effective stress reliever aids relaxation and eases breathing, as we tend to breathe in a shallow way when stressed or concentrating. Good for coughs and colds (but take care if you have asthma).

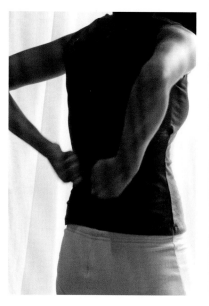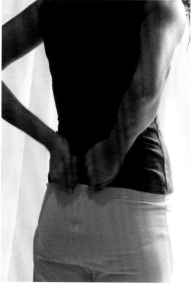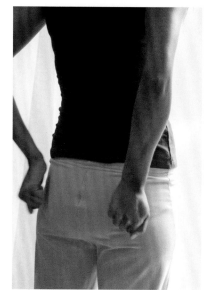

6 Make fists and gently drum-roll over the kidneys (avoid if you have a kidney disorder). Now drum roll over the middle lower back (releasing the waist muscles that work hard keeping us upright) and the buttocks to release the gluteal muscles. Now gently drum roll the backs of the legs to boost circulation. Continue on the backs of the calves and the fronts of the thighs.

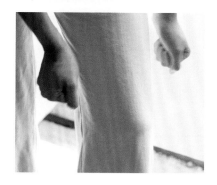

7 Rotate your left ankle to the left and then to the right three times. Now repeat with the right ankle. This is helpful if you have been wearing heels all day and need a little pick-me-up. Rise up on the balls of your feet and then lower your feet until they are flat on the ground. This releases all the muscles in the feet and massages the reflex points for the spine, as well as toning your arches. This exercise is also recommended as a foot strengthener for fallen arches.

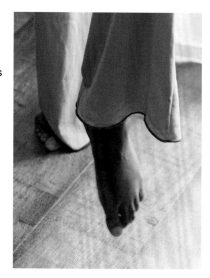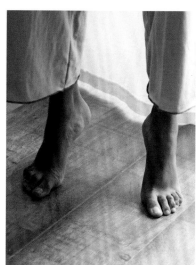

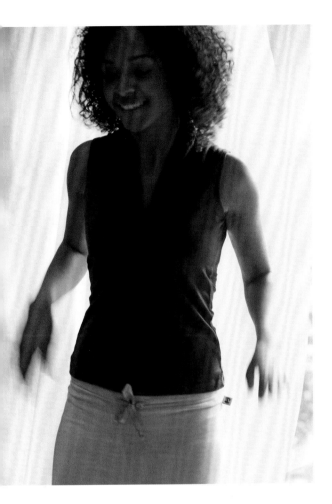

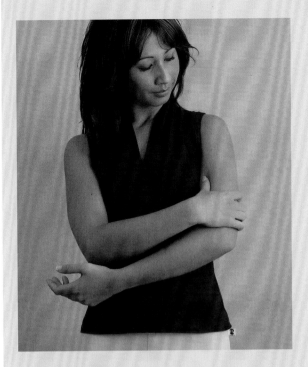

SQUEEZE AND RELEASE

This simple and effective movement is ideal as a self-massage technique when you are on the move. Use it to ease taut muscles and boost the flow of blood and lymph. It is perfect for the arms and releases tension that builds up after a tiring day. Hold your left wrist with your right hand and squeeze and release, working up your inner arm. Now repeat on your outer arm. Repeat the hand and arm sequence with your left hand working your right wrist and arm. Use a slow, rhythmic movement and keep your hands relaxed and supple. To access deeper areas of tension, use a kneading action to really work the muscle. Cup your hand over the muscle and roll it between your fingers and the heel of the hand.

8 One of my favorites. Shake all over like a Brazilian samba dancer standing "still." Shake your arms, legs, and whole body. Imagine you are a jelly wobbling on a plate. Allow all your muscles, flesh, and bones to shake and wobble. Shake your hands as if trying to dry them and move your body from right to left with your head looking from right to left. Do this for a minute or two. This is a great invigorator—you will really feel awake after doing this, and better than an espresso!

giving a massage on the move

If you're with a traveling companion or colleague, you can take turns to give each other this marvelous stress-relieving massage. Seat the recipient on a comfortable chair with the chair back to the side, so that you can access the whole of the back easily. Get them to sit with their feet hip-width apart, backs of the thighs firmly on the seat, and hands relaxed, palms downwards and resting on their thighs.

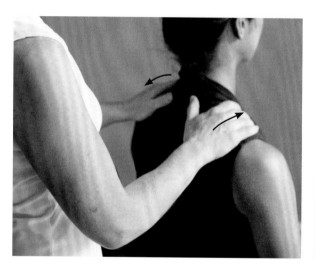

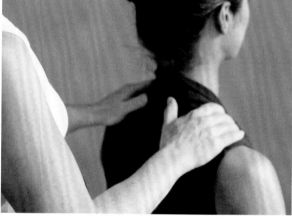

1 Place your hands on the recipient's shoulders. Keeping your hands connected to their shoulders, move their upper body from right to left with alternating movements. This is a great way to relieve stress in the shoulders—I call this the "shoulder shudder." It's also a good move to go back to during the massage to monitor progress. I always start with this move as the recipient cannot help but relax.

2 With open palms, sweep across the tops of the shoulders and down the arms. This helps the connection build between you and the recipient and also creates the sensation of sweeping away the tension of the day while relaxing the neck, shoulders, and arms. This move also helps to sweep away the energetic tension accumulated around the shoulders and arms.

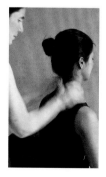
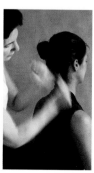
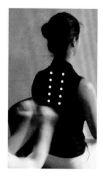

3 With open palms, pat both shoulders simultaneously. This invigorates the whole shoulder area. Now use light hammering movements, alternating right and left on the right shoulder then the left shoulder, and then all over the back. Avoid the spine or any other bony parts of the back. Spend extra time on the lower back, or any area that the recipient says feels tense. Thinking of a tune can help maintain an even tempo of movement as you drum lightly.

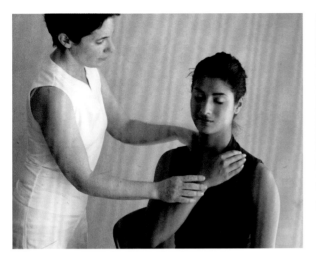

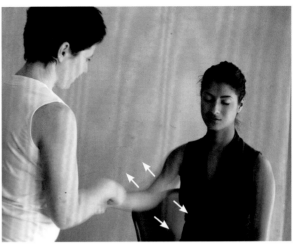

4 Stand to the side of the recipient, holding their hand against their chest to relax their arm and shoulder, and provide a firm base for you to massage against. Knead the shoulder by opening and closing your hand as if squeezing dough. Be gentle and always check they are comfortable with the pressure before massaging more deeply.

5 Hold the hand and shake the arm and then swing it from side to side. This is a great muscle and joint relaxer. Now gently massage and shake each finger. I usually keep repeating the arm "shake-out" as each time this move takes the tension relief to a deeper level.

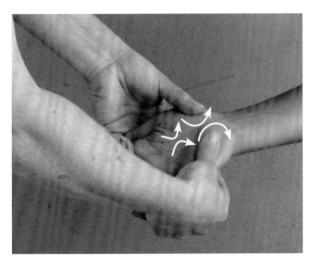

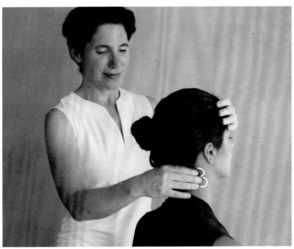

6 Spread the palm open by interlinking your little fingers with the first and little fingers of the recipient's hand and stretch. Press with your thumbs to release any tension. Repeat on the other hand. Then repeat step 1 (shoulder shudder) to assess how much tension has been released.

7 Support the head with your left hand by letting the forehead rest in the contour of your palm. Cup your right hand around the back of the neck. Begin at the ridges of the occiput and work your way down the neck, gently circling and pulling as you go. Repeat five times.

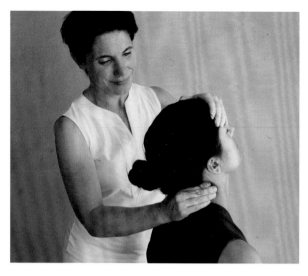

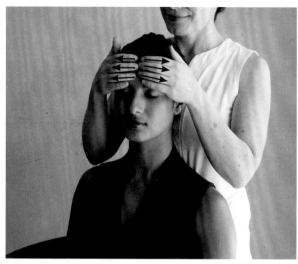

8 In the same position, rest the thumb and fingers of your right hand in the occipital ridges and support the skull as you gently push the head back with your left hand. This should be done very gently and comfortably. This helps relieve neck tension and give relief from the heavy weight of the head.

9 Standing behind the recipient now, rest their head against you and massage the front of their skull and forehead. Start with your fingertips in the middle of the forehead and use open strokes outwards.

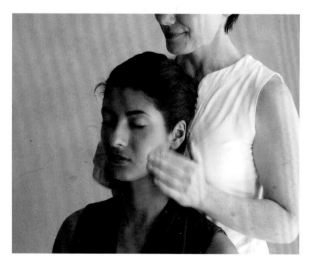

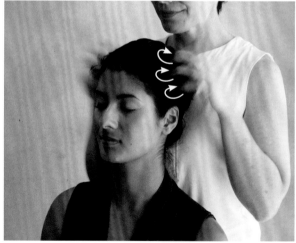

10 Rest your fingertips on the jawline and gently massage the jaw, using circular movements.

11 Now massage around the scalp, again using circular movements. Spend some time here. Remember how good it feels to have a shampoo at the hair salon. Repeat step 1 (shoulder shudder). As you do so, silently assess the changes in the recipient that have occurred so far.

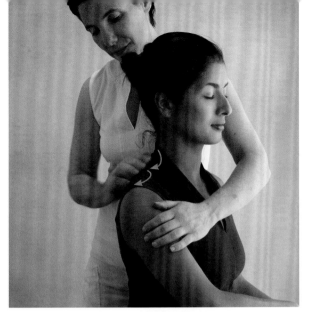

12 Massage the shoulder muscles with your fingertips. Use your right hand to massage the right shoulder, supporting the front of the recipient's right shoulder with your left. This allows you to apply comfortable pressure. Avoid massaging bony areas, such as the spine and shoulder blades. Now change position to massage the left shoulder with your left hand. Spend as much time as feels necessary. I find people love this because of the postural stresses caused by driving, computer work, and so on.

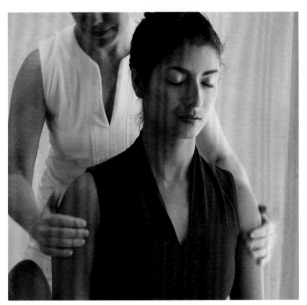

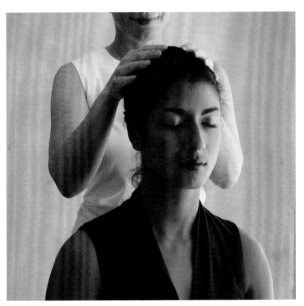

13 Now squeeze along the tops of the shoulders and down the arms. Gently squeeze along the arms, and then do the shoulder shudder (step 1) again. Now repeat any of the steps described so far until you feel you have reached a natural conclusion. This is a chance to really use your intuition. Spend some more time on any of the steps the recipient seems to really enjoy or you feel may need more attention.

14 To end the sequence, rest your hands on the top of their head. Imagine warm, liquid golden light pouring from your hands into their head, then into their shoulders, down their back, and through their legs and feet. Spend some time imagining them being grounded, alert, relaxed, and refreshed. To finish, gently lift your hands and walk away, leaving your recipient to revive slowly. Wash your hands and shake away any residual energy you may have picked up during the massage session.

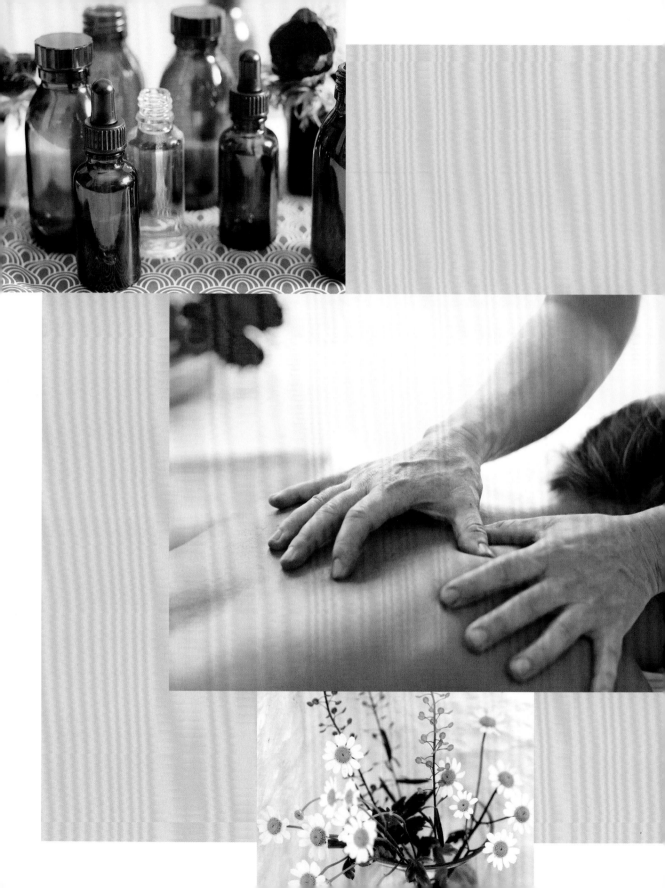

chapter 6

aromatherapy

In this chapter, I share the essential oils that I use most frequently and explain all the steps you need to blend the oils for a simple aromatherapy massage. As well as massage, these healing and uplifting oils can be used to alleviate physical and emotional symptoms in a variety of ways, from applying the oils to acupressure points to making an essential bath oil.

aromatherapy—the ancient healer

Found in Ayurveda, Traditional Chinese Medicine, and Western Herbalism, aromatherapy uses the aromatic essences of plants, flowers, and trees for healing purposes. In my practice I use 50 essential oils and have been amazed by the potent effect that essential oils have on the mind, body, and spirit. It seems that the simpler I make the mix, the more effective it is.

making a blend

Use a plant-based oil as the massage (or carrier) oil for aromatherapy blends, as mineral-based oils, such as baby oil, do not penetrate the skin. Use the following proportions of essential oil to massage oil, according to skin type.

aromatherapy massage blend

I generally use 4–8 drops of essential oil to 20–25ml of carrier oil for a massage.

For sensitive skin:
• Add up to 4 drops essential oil to 20ml carrier oil.
• Add 20 drops essential oil to 100ml carrier oil.

For normal skin:
• Add up to 8 drops essential oil to 20ml carrier oil.
• Add 40 drops essential oil to 100ml carrier oil.

topical healing blend

You can use a stronger proportion, 8–10 drops per 20ml, for a topical rub to help alleviate period pain or a chest rub for a cold (see health tips for common ailments, pages 138–141).

massage (carrier) oils

For a basic massage (or "carrier") oil I like to use a nut or seed oil such as almond or sunflower. Always check whether the recipient is allergic to nuts, and use grapeseed or sunflower instead. Whenever possible, go for organic, cold-pressed oil. Carrier oils mixed with a few drops of essential oil transport the essential oil into the body and help it last longer by slowing down its evaporation. Never apply essential oils directly to the skin as they are highly concentrated and may cause irritation. Choose from the following light, medium, or rich oils for massage:

light	medium	rich
soya	sweet almond	sesame
holly	coconut	avocado
sunflower	grapeseed	jojoba

If you like, you can also add the following specialist oils to any blend: wheatgerm, for its moisturizing properties and its vitamin E content, which can aid aging, dry or sun-damaged skin, and calendula, to soften scar tissue and treat inflamed/cracked skin.

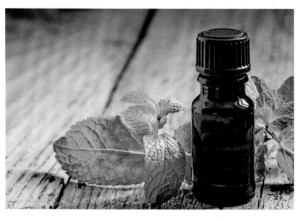

essential oil profiles

Here are nine essential oils that I use frequently because they have the widest range of actions. They will make a good basis for your personal aromatherapy kit and a wide variety of blends.

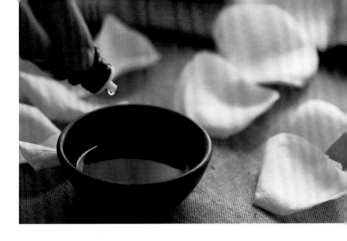

bergamot *(citrus bergamia)*

Bergamot is the essence that gives Earl Grey tea its distinctive flavor. It eases tension and is the perfect oil to combat the stresses and frustrations of life.

emotional aspects Bergamot helps to release pent-up emotions and a sense of being "stuck" in your life. It alleviates feelings of irritability, frustration, and anger, especially when one's plans are continually thwarted. It has an uplifting and lightening quality, promoting a sense of liberation. Bergamot relieves anxiety and angry depression and helps alleviate addictive urges. It is a perfect oil to add to any blend after a stressful day juggling office, travel, and home.

physical aspects Bergamot is the ideal oil to treat irritable bowel syndrome (IBS), migraine, and tension headaches, especially affecting the eyes, as well as mild asthma, premenstrual syndrome (PMS), and dysmenorrhea (painful periods). It can be added to cold and flu remedies to aid relaxation, thereby enhancing healing and recovery. It also treats oily skin conditions, such as acne and seborrhea.

cedarwood *(cedrus atlantica)*

The name cedrus originates from the Arabic word "kedron," meaning power. Its woody, musky notes make us feel grounded, and yet elevated with a renewed sense of willpower. Cedarwood bolsters the kidneys and enhances general energy levels, seeming to give the strength and rootedness of the tree itself.

emotional aspects Cedarwood reinforces one's sense of identity and boundaries. It eases feelings of alienation, and so is perfect to use on business trips, or before exams, interviews, or presentations. It helps remind you who you really are when the touchstones of your identity, such as home, partner or friends, are not around. It keeps you grounded and rooted—ideal when starting a new job or endeavor. It aids recovery after prolonged stress, alleviates depression due to fear, fatigue, or exhaustion, and is a powerful emotional support and confidence booster.

physical aspects Cedarwood boosts general energy. It relieves backache and urogenital problems and helps recovery after periods of insomnia, helping one regain strength and stamina. Through its action on the kidneys, cedarwood counteracts fluid retention. It has an astringent quality, ideal for oily skin and hairs and also helps recovery from hair loss caused by prolonged, stress, fear, or grief.

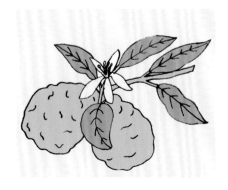

chamomile (roman)
(chamaemelum nobile)

Chamomile essential oil has a wide range of actions that simply and quickly calm the body, mind, and heart.

emotional aspects Chamomile restores emotional balance and dispels anxiety. It aids restful sleep, even in children, and so can calm a fractious child. It is this gentle, calming action that makes it perfect for adults, too. It eases irritability, feelings of anger, and nervous tension, and the depression that can arise after long periods of feeling unsupported.

physical aspects Chamomile relieves stomach cramps due to nervous tension, anticipatorial anxiety, or anger. Its anti-inflammatory qualities are useful for general pain relief, period pain, headache, earache, and toothache. It can calm skin inflammation, itching, boils, insect bites, and rashes, especially those due to allergies. I also recommend chamomile for hay fever.

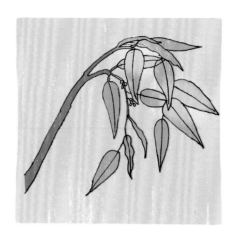

eucalyptus *(eucalyptus globulus)*

There are over 300 varieties of eucalyptus. I have chosen this one as it is the most popular and readily available. Its main action is on the respiratory system as a decongestant. It is the best cold and flu remedy.

emotional aspects As it has a strong action on the lungs, it helps us let go of the past by breathing out the old and breathing in the new, releasing thoughts that stop us living in the "now." It fortifies us after a bereavement, giving a feeling of expansion and courage to accept new experiences.

physical aspects As a decongestant, it is perfect for cold or flu symptoms, and for sinusitis, bronchitis, and mild asthma. I find a simple steam bath with a few drops of eucalyptus, tea tree and lavender in a basin with a towel over my head is as effective now as when I was a child. A powerful support to the immune system, this anti-viral oil also helps fight off colds and flu, and is effective in the treatment of cold sores when applied directly with a cotton bud (along with tea tree). Blended with lemon essential oil, it is an effective insect repellent, but do not use neat.

CAUTION
Do not use if you have epilepsy.

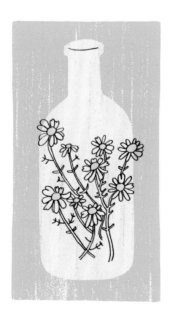

geranium *(pelargonium graveolens)*

In English folklore, geranium was used to attract a lover and aid sexual fulfillment. It supports the feminine aspect, helping us connect with our intuition, instincts, and the joy of life. It is perfect for those who have lost touch with their liberated, sensual, or creative side after a prolonged period of hard work or responsibility.

emotional aspects Geranium is a useful addition to a healing blend for anyone suffering depression or anxiety due to stress from overwork or other reasons out of their control. It is the perfect antidote for those who have lost touch with the "real world" outside work. Its refreshingly sweet scent stimulates the senses, renewing our sense of joy, earthly wonder, and simple creativity, and calms the heart and mind. I often use it to treat the mood swings of PMS.

physical aspects Geranium alleviates breast tenderness in PMS and menopausal symptoms, such as hot flushes, night sweats, red cheeks, depression, anxiety, and mood swings. It is effective for dry and inflamed skin conditions, too, such as itchy dry dermatitis. It relieves headaches due to mental or physical fatigue and promotes a healthy balance of work, rest, creativity, sensuality, and play.

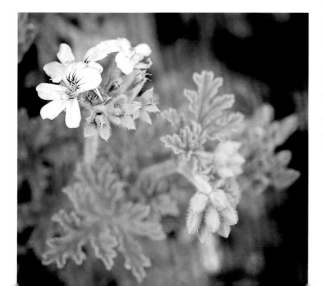

ginger *(zingiber officinale)*

Ginger has been used in Traditional Chinese and Ayurvedic medicine for centuries as a warming and strengthening ingredient. When I lived in Malaysia, local midwives told me that new mothers eat Ginger Chicken (chicken cooked with vegetables and fresh slices of ginger) for 40 days after childbirth to help the uterus contract quickly and easily as well as building up the strength of the mother after the depleting effects of pregnancy and childbirth.

emotional aspects Ginger's positive effect on emotions mainly comes from its ability to strengthen the body physically, boosting vitality. It is great for those who need a boost to complete (or begin!) an important project. It enhances the libido and trust in one's own physical prowess. According to Chinese medicine, ginger boosts the kidney Chi, so enhancing willpower and personal resolve. In Ayurveda, ginger raises the energy of the root chakra (see page 46).

physical aspects Ginger can be used to treat any kind of physical debility or pain, especially muscular pain due to overuse, or excessive cold leading to cramping pain. It eases period pain, and abdominal pain and swelling due to IBS, overeating, or trapped wind. I recommend tea made with fresh ginger for colds and flu. Peel and slice a thumb's length of fresh ginger, and steep in boiling water for five minutes. Add lemon, honey, and cinnamon. This warming tea, taken in winter, can boost energy and so prevent colds and flu. Ginger also helps physical and nervous exhaustion due to periods of stress, hard work, or illness, and is a great remedy for travel sickness and nausea.

CAUTION
Do not use if you are pregnant or have high blood pressure.

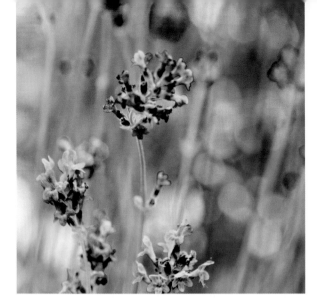

lavender (alpine)
(lavendula angustifolia)

Lavender is one oil I would not be without. It has the widest action of all oils, emotionally and physically. It is an effective oil to calm the emotions and treat stress. Lavender is strongly antiseptic and makes an ideal wound and burn healer, promoting rapid tissue repair and guarding against infection. In Europe it is traditionally used as a general disinfectant, as well as to "welcome" the baby and soothe the mother.

emotional aspects My favorite is Alpine lavender, which seems to encapsulate the vast quiet stillness of the mountains. Lavender is a great oil to use if you feel overwhelmed or oversensitive. It helps calm irritability, anger, and hot-headed behavior and so genuinely helps us "be cool." As well as effectively alleviating anxiety and depression, it helps you relax and unwind, especially for those who cannot stop long enough to rest and recuperate, no matter how tired. Lavender is also good for mild shock—the equivalent of Dr Bach's Flower Rescue Remedy.

physical aspects Lavender is a highly effective burn treatment. René Gattefosse, a 19th-century French scientist, "discovered" modern aromatherapy after plunging his hand into a vat of lavender oil to cool a burn. He was amazed at how it quickly relieved the inflammation, and the wound healed with little scarring. I always keep lavender handy in case of burns—after running the burn under very cold water, I use lavender essential oil with ice-cold water pads to cool the wound further and then apply the oil directly to the skin and put a cold compress on top. Lavender also relieves sunburn, perfect when mixed with aloe vera gel. It reduces inflammation and relieves itching, and is ideal for itchy or infected insect bites, and acne. It is good for all kinds of pain, including muscular aches, and also lowers blood pressure. Lavender is the best remedy for headaches due to tension or arguments, and aids restful sleep. I would not be without it.

CAUTION
Do not use during the first three months of pregnancy.

rosemary *(rosemarinus officinalis)*

Rosemary has been used throughout the centuries in Ancient Egypt and Greece as an herb of remembrance to commemorate the dead. In England it has a long history as a potent medicinal herb. Rosemary has a wide range of actions that benefit mind and body. It is a warming and strengthening oil that increases our mental agility, focus and memory, as well as fortifying all the body's organs. "Seethe much Rosemary," said William Langham, in *The Garden of Health* (1597), "and bathe therein to make thee lusty, lively, joyfull, likeing and youngly."

emotional aspects An exhilarating oil, rosemary instills enthusiasm and restores faith in our innate potential. It can enhance memory and relieve apathy and mental fatigue, and so is a great study aid as well as reviving and refreshing the mind after periods of intense intellectual activity. Rosemary's ability to fortify the heart and increase zest for life can help us become enlivened by life and is a powerful antidote to lethargy and gloom. This herb of remembrance helps us recall those lost to us, and our true passions, dreams, and potential. I use rosemary for those who lose hope of recovery after a long period of illness. It helps give strength and the belief that they can recuperate.

physical aspects Rosemary is a powerful physical tonic for the whole body. It strengthens the heart, spleen, liver, kidneys, and musculature. It eases headaches due to exhaustion, lack of sleep, or excess mental effort, it boosts mental stamina and enlivens the mind. Rosemary alleviates muscle tension, stiffness, and pain, especially in the back and limbs, and strengthens physical weakness of any kind. It boosts the blood circulation, thereby treating cold hands and feet. Women used to rinse their hair in rosemary water to give it shine and also fortify their mind, especially as they grew older! To avoid skin irritation, use no more than two drops in a bath or massage.

CAUTION
Do not use if you are pregnant or have high blood pressure or epilepsy.

with earthy notes, helps you get back in touch with your truest nature and provides a buffer against the pressures and desires of others. Thought to help promote a connection with the divine, it helps re-affirm your identity and connection with your higher self. Burn sandalwood incense or combine with frankincense to make a meditation blend and put a few drops on your pulse points and third eye (see chakras, pages 44–48).

physical aspects Sandalwood treats urinary tract infections, such as cystitis, and the back pain often associated with them. It can relieve burning digestive conditions such as ulcers or diarrhea and is a useful treatment for chest infections when the mucus is yellow or green (which according to Traditional Chinese Medicine shows signs of excess heat). It makes a wonderful insect repellent and has been used to protect fine silks and other rich materials from moths. Sandalwood's cooling and drying effect treats itchy, weeping skin conditions such as "wet" eczema.

sandalwood *(santalum album)*

Sandalwood has long been associated with spiritual life. It instills a sense of mental calmness and focus, helping you acquire the quiet insight needed to gain the full benefit of meditation. For this reason, many temples and religious icons in India were made of sandalwood and its incense is still burned during Buddhist and Hindu rituals today. It is a calming essential oil that dries and cools.

emotional aspects Sandalwood cools and eases agitation, worry, and irritability, calms the mind, and stills chattering thoughts. Its heady scent, infused

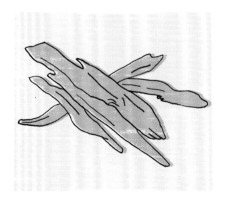

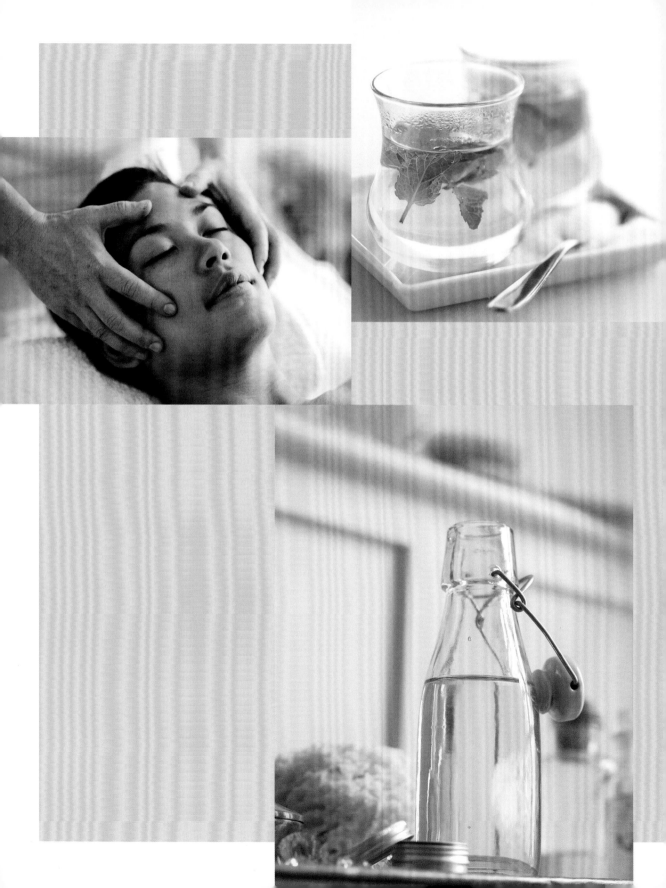

natural remedies

On the following pages, you will find health tips and advice for targeting many common ailments, from physical aches and pains to the common cold. This holistic approach draws on many of the techniques described in this book, from Ayurveda and aromatherapy to reflexology, acupressure, and, of course, massage, to speed up healing and bring harmony and balance to body, mind, and soul.

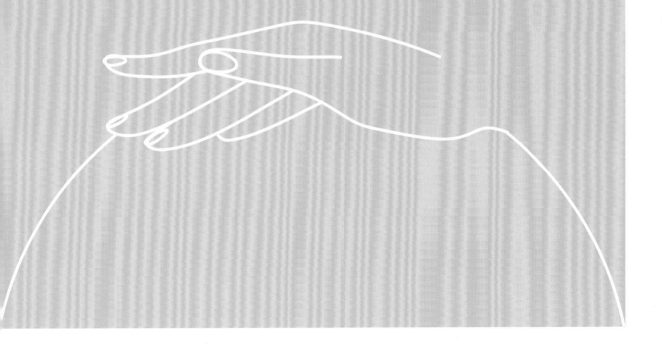

health tips for common ailments

This holistic advice draws on all the techniques described in this book—techniques from both East and West, ancient and modern—to aid relaxation and restoration in the targeted areas where you need it most.

head and face

headache

massage: Add two drops of an essential oil to a tablespoon of carrier oil; massage into the neck and head (page 130). Use bergamot for headache around the forehead with irritability, lavender for general headache with eye pain and feeling overwhelmed, and rosemary for headache with tiredness and lack of mental clarity.

acupressure: Activate acupoints LI–4, Liv–3, GB–1 (pages 100, 104, 108).

reflexology: Massage big toe point (pages 36–38).

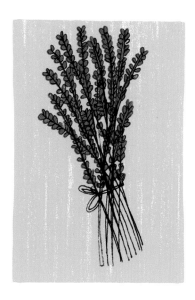

earache

aromatherapy: Open a small ball of cotton wool and add a drop of chamomile essential oil. Close the cotton ball tightly and place gently in the ear.

acupressure: Activate acupoint GB–20 (page 109).

eyestrain

prevention: Take a break every 45 minutes from the computer, read in plenty of light, and do this exercise: Look at a nearby object and then one farther away. Repeat five times. Regularly look at the horizon.

herbal: Brew two chamomile teabags in a mug of boiling water, cool and squeeze out. Lie comfortably and place the teabags on your eyelids for ten minutes. You can also refrigerate the tea—saturate cotton pads with tea, then use as an eye mask.

acupressure: Activate acupoint GB–20 (page 109).

sinus congestion

traditional chinese medicine: Reduce phlegm and mucus production by avoiding food containing wheat, dairy foods, and sugar. Avoid oranges and orange juice.

aromatherapy: Make a facial steam bath: Fill a bowl or basin with hot water; add a drop each of eucalyptus, lavender, and tea tree essential oils. Lean over the bowl, cover your head with a towel, and breathe gently.

massage: Using the simple massage sequence shown in step 4 on page 23, massage around the sinus area.

acupressure: Activate acupoint Lu–7 (page 101).

spots and pimples

traditional chinese medicine: If the skin is generally red, with raised red bumps or yellow heads, the tongue is red with a dry or yellow coat, and there is a feeling of frustration, the cause is too much heat. Apply organic rose or lavender water. Eat fresh fruit and vegetables (no oranges, tomatoes, eggplant, and bananas), and avoid alcohol, wheat, sugar, red meat, and spicy foods. If the complexion is pale, with blackheads or raised white lumps with white heads, the tongue is pale, wet, and swollen, and there is a feeling of tiredness, the cause is excess cold. Drink herbal tea made with fresh rosemary leaves. Eat warming foods such as fresh vegetable soup and avoid ice cream, cold fizzy drinks, sugary foods, and dairy products.

aromatherapy: Have a daily facial steam bath, for excess cold type person—not recommended for over-heated skin (see sinus congestion for method) and add a drop each of rosemary and tea tree essential oils, then wipe the skin with lavender water.

reflexology: For a couple of minutes each day, massage the facial reflexology point on top of the big toe, starting beneath the toenail (pages 36–38).

acupressure: Activate acupoint GV–26 (page 109).

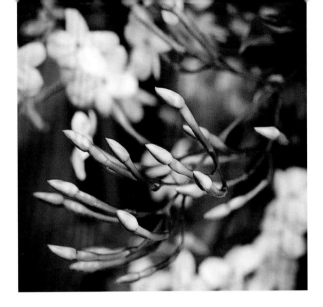

neck, torso, and abdomen

sore throat

aromatherapy: Add sea salt and a drop each of lavender, clary sage, and tea tree essential oils to warm water, mix well, and gargle (do not swallow).

herbal: Add a teaspoon of dried sage to a cup of boiling water, cover, steep for five minutes, then strain, leave to cool, and use to gargle.

ayurveda: Add a pinch of turmeric and a dash of honey to warm milk and gargle—or drink if you like.

acupressure: Activate acupoint Li–4 (page 100).

colds

traditional chinese medicine: For a cold accompanied by sweating, fever, yellow mucus, or a very dry cough and general heat, make a facial steam bath (see sinus congestion for method) and add a drop each of lavender, lemon, eucalyptus (citriadora) essential oils. Or add a drop of each oil to a tablespoon of carrier oil and massage into the chest and sinus area.

herbal: Drink ginger tea: Cut a thumb-size piece of fresh ginger, peel and slice, and steep in a cup of boiling water for at least five minutes, then add a little honey (to taste) and a slice of lemon.

acupressure: Activate acupoints LI–4 (page 100) to unblock sinuses and relieve headache; Lu–1 (page 106) to boost lung energy and clear chest; Liv–3 (page 104), if feeling irritable.

irritable bowel syndrome

prevention: Make mealtime a calm, pleasurable experience. Eat in a relaxed, unhurried way, chewing your food slowly and carefully until it is completely broken down. Avoid eating fruit with other food—allow an hour before or after meals.

ayurveda: Don't drink water with meals—allow 20 minutes afterwards. (The fire element is an important part of digestion and water would dampen the fire.) Avoid cigarette smoke, tea, coffee, wheat, and excess sugary foods. Wear loose, comfortable clothes and avoid wearing constricting clothes or tights.

massage: Make a blend of bergamot and chamomile in a carrier oil and rub into your abdomen.

acupressure: Activate acupoints GB–34 and St–25 (pages 103 and 106).

menstrual pain

massage: For menstruation accompanied by feelings of moodiness, irritability, cramping pain, and light to medium menstrual flow, blend clary sage, chamomile, and bergamot with a carrier oil |and massage the abdomen. For menstruation accompanied by tearfulness, cramping pain, and a heavy menstrual flow, blend jasmine, lavender, cypress, and chamomile with a carrier oil and massage the abdomen.

acupressure: Activate acupoints Liv–2 (page 103) and Sp–6 (page 104).

professional help: For deep-rooted problems try a long-term course of acupuncture or reflexology.

lower body

lower backache

massage: For general backache, blend a drop each of rosemary, ginger, and lavender oils with carrier oil and massage into the lower back (page 17–18).

acupressure: Activate acupoints Bl–23 and GB–30 (page 110–111).

professional help: For chronic backache, see a professional aromatherapist, cranial/sacral osteopath, or acupressurist/acupuncturist.

CAUTION

If back pain is felt constantly around the kidney area (just below waist level), see a doctor.

lack of sex drive

aromatherapy massage: For lowered libido due to stress and exhaustion, mix one drop each of ginger, rosemary, bergamot, and ylang ylang in a tablespoon of massage oil and rub into the lower back and chest.

Traditional Chinese Medicine: Drink fresh ginger tea (see colds for method). Kidneys are the seat of our energy and ginger is a kidney tonic that will pep up general energy levels as well as libido. Take walks in the fresh air, improve your diet, and take a good-quality vitamin supplement. Dance and listen to music.

acupressure: Activate acupoints Ki–6 (page 105), Bl–23 (page 110) and Ht–3 (page 102).

fertility support

professional help: For both partners, have a course of reflexology, ayurvedic massage, and panacha karma (a cleanse and treatment to balance the Doshas), or acupuncture and Chinese herbs.

diet and lifestyle: Eat fresh fruit and vegetables, and avoid caffeine, alcohol, and excess sugar. I suggest you take folic acid supplements (1mg per day) or a good, pre-natal vitamin supplement for three months before you plan to conceive or as soon as you know you are pregnant. Take plenty of gentle exercise.

acupressure: Activate acupoints Ki–6 (page 105) and CV–4 (page 107).

dry skin

massage: Make a moisturizing blend of four drops of geranium, two tablespoons of avocado oil, and two tablespoons of almond oil. Massage into your skin while damp. Allow the oil to sink in before dressing.

diet: Include more olive oil, almonds, Brazil nuts, and cashews in your diet and take a vitamin E or evening primrose oil supplement. Drink lots of water and avoid coffee, colas, and alcohol.

athlete's foot

prevention: Avoid yeast and sugar. Drink more water. Wear cotton socks and dry your feet carefully after a shower or bath using a separate towel.

aromatherapy: Make a foot soak: Dissolve sea salt crystals in hot water. Add cold water to cool plus

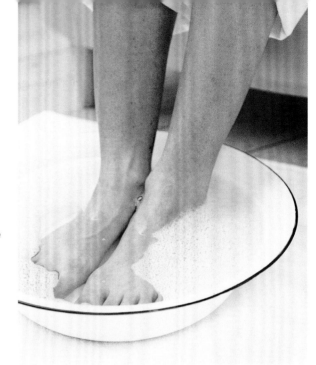

three drops of tea tree and two drops of lavender essential oils. Dry your feet and gently massage in a blend of one tablespoon almond oil and three drops of tea tree oil and allow to sink in before dressing.

verruca

aromatherapy: Add two drops each of tea tree, thyme, and lemon essential oils to 2fl oz (50ml) of tincture of thuja (available from an herbal dispensary) and dab onto the verruca using a cotton bud. Cover with a sticking plaster. Alternatively, just add a drop of tea tree or lemon essential oil to a cotton bud and dab on.

traditional: Peel a fresh garlic clove; slice in half. Place on the verruca and cover with a plaster.

professional: See a medical herbalist if the verruca does not clear up in a few weeks. Herbal tinctures taken internally may rid the body of the verruca virus.

index

resources

recommended reading:

Aromatherapy for Healing the Spirit, Gabriel Mojay (Gaia Books, 2005)

Ayurveda: The Science of Self-Healing, Dr Vasant Lad (Lotus Press, 1984)

Between Heaven and Earth: A Guide to Chinese Medicine, Harriet Beinfeld & Efrem Korngold (Ballantine Books, 1992)

Care of the Soul, Thomas Moore (Piatakus Books, 1992)

The Foundations of Chinese Medicine: A Comprehensive Text for Acupuncturists and Herbalists, (Churchill Livingstone, 1989)

Hands of Light: A Guide to Healing Through the Human Energy Field, Barbara Ann Brennan (Bantam 1988)

Healing with Qualities: The Essence of Time Therapy, Manuel Schoch (Sentient Publications, 2004)

Simply Ayurveda: Discover Your Type to Transform Your Life, Bharti Vyas (Thorsons, 2000)

Women's Bodies Women's Wisdom: The Complete Guide to Women's Health and Wellbeing, Christiane Northrup MD (Piatkus Books, 1998)

recommended websites:

International Federation of Professional Aromatherapists (IFPA) and Gabriel Moray
www.aromatherapy-studies.com

Association of Reflexologists (AOR)
www.aor.org.uk

www.daphneroubini.ca

Model's clothing, pages 112–127: Sweaty Betty.
www.sweatybetty.com

acknowledgments

the author wishes to thank: Gabriel Mojay for his generosity of spirit and my original training in Oriental Aromatherapy and bodywork. Manuel Schoch for sharing his authenticity, and the "loving mediation" with me. Peter Lim for my apprenticeship in The Rwo-Shur health method. Colleen Fraser of The Vida wellness Spa and Whistler Healing Arts for the Ayurvedic questionnaire and sharing her knowledge of Ayurveda with me. Andrew Flower for his support over the years and casting an eye over the acupressure chapter. Arthur Molinary for his down-to-earth tuition. The publisher Cindy Richards and the talented team at CICO Books. Liz Dean for her great editorial input, support, and hilarious friendship. Tino Tedaldi and Jo for their hard work and great job shooting the photos, Christine Wood for the beautiful design, Richard Emerson for his skillful editorial input, Andrew Smith for the love and joy he brings to my life, and Jeni Couzyn for her revelations and laughter. To Fe and Catherine for the many years. Jill for sea wall walks and chats. And to my mum, Esther Roubini, the first person ever to massage me.

picture credits: